"The creative and brilliantly wired mind of scientist and author Dr. Ski Chilton again boldly explores human behavior potential in his insightful latest book, *The ReWired Brain*—a provocative mental journey."

Charles (Cash) McCall, MD, professor of translational science and molecular medicine, Wake Forest University School of Medicine

"Change—honest, God-honoring change—is difficult! It seems at times the Christian community oscillates between two extremes: religious denial or the insanity of just trying harder to be better. *The ReWired Brain* instead gives hope and practical insights into how we can get 'unstuck' in life. Using engaging insights from Scripture, neuroscience, and the author's personal struggles, the reader is drawn into the great adventure of becoming like Christ. The book is a rich tapestry of fascinating analogies from contemporary literature, film, and current events that assist the reader in understanding the dynamics of renewing your mind through 'rewiring.' Having spent over thirty years counseling pastors and Christian leaders who were seriously trapped in life, I would strongly recommend this creative contribution to the battle for wholeness and holiness."

Dr. Ted Roberts, bestselling author, pastor, and certified sexual addiction counselor

THE
REWIRED
BRAIN

FREE YOURSELF *of* NEGATIVE BEHAVIORS
and RELEASE YOUR BEST SELF

DR. SKI CHILTON

WITH **DR. MARGARET RUKSTALIS** AND **A. J. GREGORY**

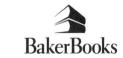

BakerBooks

a division of Baker Publishing Group
Grand Rapids, Michigan

Published by Baker Books
a division of Baker Publishing Group
P.O. Box 6287, Grand Rapids, MI 49516-6287
www.bakerbooks.com

Printed in the United States of America

Library of Congress Cataloging-in-Publication Data
Names: Chilton, Floyd H., author.
Title: The reWired brain : free yourself of negative behaviors and release your best self / Dr. Ski
    Chilton, with Dr. Margaret Rukstalis and A.J. Gregory.
Description: Grand Rapids : Baker Books, 2016. | Includes bibliographical references.
Identifiers: LCCN 2016006233 | ISBN 9780801007477 (cloth)
Subjects: LCSH: Thought and thinking—Religious aspects—Christianity.
Classification: LCC BV4598.4 .C45 2016 | DDC 158.1—dc23
LC record available at https://lccn.loc.gov/2016006233

ISBN 9780801019463

The author is represented by The FEDD Agency, Inc.

22   23   24   25   26   8   7   6

Contents

Introduction

Growing up in a small tobacco farming community at the foothills of the Appalachian Mountains in North Carolina did not stir much excitement. But when Daddy brought home our first black-and-white television set, it was like the second coming. Outfitted with rabbit-ear antennas, it occupied a corner of our tiny two-room cinderblock house. Because my family lived in the backwoods, not even having the luxury of indoor plumbing, the only channel we could get was CBS. Just as well. It was the one network that broadcasted an annual showing of my favorite movie, *The Wizard of Oz*.

Waiting year after year for that brilliant film to air was like waiting for the president's arrival. My parents, my sister, and I would huddle around the set in the small living room, which also served as the bedroom to us all, in great anticipation, as if we had never before seen the film. While the movie is dear to me for several reasons, fifty years later I am struck by its brilliant message that, all throughout their perilous adventure, Dorothy and her pals had always possessed the very things they were desperately seeking. Dorothy could go home at any time. The Scarecrow already had a brain, the Tin Man a heart, and the Lion courage. And yet they were convinced that the Wizard was the only one who could remedy all of their problems.

The scene in which Dorothy and her entourage finally arrive in Oz and stand before the great and powerful Wizard still gives me chills. Seeing his giant head shrouded in smoke and flames and carrying on in a booming and threatening voice frightened the living daylights out of me as a child. But as we all discovered, there was nothing to be afraid of. The great and powerful Wizard didn't exist, just a wise little man behind the curtain.

I love the scene near the end when the Tin Man asks Dorothy what she learned in Oz. She responds, "Well, I—I think that it—that it wasn't enough to just want to see Uncle Henry and Auntie Em—and it's that if I ever go looking for my heart's desire again, I won't look any farther than my own backyard. Because if it isn't there, I never lost it to begin with!"[1]

Like Dorothy, many of us are lost in the inner dimensions of our minds, trying to discover who we are and why we are here. We wander through a wilderness of bewildering and difficult places, situations, and relationships. Perhaps most menacing are the cyclones of our past experiences, such as traumatic childhoods, critical broken relationships, and difficult life transitions, which produce in us fear, shame, anxiety, and depression.

What would happen if you discovered you have within you the capacity to heal your past brokenness, to direct the transformation of your mind and your life? What would happen if you finally realized you have more power over your unhealthy behaviors, painful feelings, and harmful interactions than you think? What would happen if you realized the past devastation and current chaos of your life could become the critical lessons necessary to move you to a higher state of consciousness? What would happen if you could unleash the power of your mind to live your best life?

What This Book Offers

Great news! As human beings, we have the capacity through our incredibly powerful and flexible minds to transport ourselves back to Kansas. Should we choose, we can transition our lives from discontent and static to beauty and joy. Through science, psychology, and real-life stories, *The Re-Wired Brain* will help you understand the framework of your mind. You will be able to determine the reason you continue to engage in destructive behaviors and have such negative feelings. You will learn how to recognize harmful emotional patterns and how to stop engaging in them. And you will be able to do all of this through the plasticity (flexibility) of your brain and your enormous and wonderful capacity to rewire it.

This book focuses on the human brain because it serves as the foundation, hardware, and software for all of our reactions, responses, behaviors, emotions, sensations, and choices. It is the source of millions of unconscious and a far smaller number of conscious thoughts each day. It is the foundational setting where we can either become and stay imprisoned in unhappiness or discover and live in freedom. To move forward, we must venture into our brains and reexamine our lives to make sense of our past and current actions, recognize our faulty and destructive habits and patterns, and ultimately rewire them so we can have joyful and meaningful lives.

In the pages that follow, you are going to read some fancy scientific and psychological terms like *brain plasticity*, *epigenetics*, and *dual process reasoning*. Don't let this language trip you up. By understanding the human brain, you are going to see how your thoughts and brain circuitry affect your emotional and spiritual journeys with God and with others.

It is not my mission to give you a technical description of how your brain works for science's sake but to allow you to name and give context for your behaviors and emotions. What you will learn is fundamental to helping you experience the process of change and find ultimate freedom in all areas of your life, including personal growth, relationships, and sexuality.

With that said, the key premise of this book is that your brain is divided into two systems of thinking (System 1 and System 2), and they compete for your attention, feelings, emotions, and actions. Supremacy by System 1 gives rise to a person who is absolutely controlled by their unconscious fears and instincts and is highly influenced by experiences from their childhood and environmental factors (such as fear-based advertisements, twenty-four-hour news cycles, and certain forms of religion). The second force or system of thinking is much more developed, deliberative, and uniquely human and where we find the true nature of a person.

Individually, these two systems of thinking are not all bad or all good, like an angel sitting on one shoulder and the devil on the other. The two simply have different roles, and both are necessary for your survival and happiness. When the two are not balanced, however, and one force dominates your thought patterns, your human experience gets compromised in meaningful and agonizing ways. No need for details here; I tell you everything about these two systems in chapter 1. What you need to know right now is that throughout this book Dr. Rukstalis and I show how you can rewire the very brain circuits from which these two forces come. She and I combine our professional and life experiences to bring you the insight provided in this book. This insight comes from my three decades of studies in biology, biochemistry, genetics (most recently epigenetics), neuroscience, philosophy, and theology at academic centers such as Wake Forest and Johns Hopkins as well as Dr. Rukstalis's three decades of study in addiction psychology at Dartmouth, Harvard, Penn, and Wake Forest universities.

What You Will Find

The ReWired Brain is broken up into three parts: Reflect, Reframe, and Rewire.

Part 1 (Reflect) explores dual process reasoning (DPR): where it comes from, why it matters, and what happens when one system veers into overdrive. Part 2 (Reframe) delves more deeply into how we can balance these two powerful systems in our brains in specific aspects of life. Part 3 (Rewire) will help you work through self-exploratory and transformational exercises and practices to rewire your brain.

At the end of each chapter in parts 1 and 2, we will ask you to thoughtfully answer some questions to help you begin the process of self-discovery and brain rewiring. Don't let these inquiries intimidate or overwhelm you. We present them as initial exercises to help you personify and activate the processes of reflection and recognition necessary for change.

This book is for you if:

- You have experienced intense pain and trauma as a result of your past.
- You have made relational mistakes that have hurt yourself and others.
- You are ready to transition away from your destructive responses and situations to find joy and peace.
- You are determined to uncover new and better ways to find and express who you really are at your core.

What This Means to Me

Before you read this book, you should know two things about me. First, I am a serious scientist who insists on using the scientific method to examine specific questions that can be addressed by science. I am also quite cognizant that the world of scientifically answerable questions is relatively small when compared to the big questions of who we are, why we are here, and whether there is a God who loves us. When we get to these issues, science cannot speak with anything near a definitive voice, and so we then must move to other disciplines such as philosophy and theology as well as our individual belief systems.

Most scientists and philosophers maintain a materialist belief system. Their central thesis is that our thoughts, our morality, our consciousness, our experiences, the partners we select, and whether we choose to believe (or not) in a higher power are products of a predetermined, complex set of chemical and electrical processes and reactions that take place in the deep recesses of our brains.

I, however, believe there is a God, what some might call a higher power, who loves and desires to interact with us. I also believe he created the extremely complex portions of our brains in order for us to be able to commune with him spiritually. It is certainly not necessary for you to share this belief to benefit from this book, but this is the place where I reside.

Second, although I have had incredible professional success in academia at both Johns Hopkins and Wake Forest Universities Schools of Medicine, as an author of four popular diet books, and as a businessman starting several profitable companies, the significant relational disasters, intense personal pain, and unexpected tragedies I have experienced in life have taught me the most. I have spent intense effort and engaged in much professional counseling trying to understand the whys of my life. The intense desire to make sense of my own reality drove me to examine the mysteries of the human brain. It prompted me ultimately to find a model that helped me understand my reality and, perhaps most importantly, the inconsistencies in my behavior. Researching through the model of our two systems of thinking helped me understand how, on the one hand, I could be this well-adjusted scientist and humanitarian who loved everyone and wanted nothing more than to make the world a better place and, on the other hand, this highly emotional, reactive, depressed, and destructive mess who kept failing at relationships and hurting himself and others no matter how he wanted to do otherwise.

Over the past decade, I have put in the hard work necessary not only to gain new understandings from the fields of neuroscience, philosophy, and psychology but also, more importantly, to get to know myself, recognize my major unconscious fears and feelings and their origins in my past, and figure out how not to react to their prompting. Most of all, I have been able to connect with God and understand that he wants nothing more than for me to experience freedom, joy, and love.

In his beautiful book *Warrior of the Light*, Paulo Coelho describes the pain and disappointments of life as "the beloved marks and scars that will open the gates of Paradise to me."[2] I love this because if we allow whatever pain we experience—whether self-inflicted or caused by others—to be our teacher, it can transition us to a new place. So if you have opened this book and are hurting at this moment, congratulations! You now have a great opportunity for the change and rewiring necessary to move you toward a better life.

We want to introduce you to your true self, perhaps for the first time, and help you be free. There is hope. There is possibility. You can experience liberty in your emotional and spiritual health, your relationships, and even your intimacy and sexual desire. It will take knowledge and courage. It will also take honest and fearless self-reflection. It will take surrender and forgiveness. It will take time. And it will take effort. But you will never again have to be stuck in a matrix of unhealthy and harmful cycles. A hopeful future of possibility awaits.

PART 1

REFLECT

We begin by taking you on a journey to get to know your brain—particularly your two systems of thinking and how they constantly battle for your attention. You will learn what happens when these two forces are not balanced and one dominates the other. By the end of this section, you will be encouraged by the exciting news that regardless of how your brain has been wired to control your behaviors and emotions thus far, it can be changed.

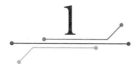

A Tale of Two Minds

> Humans are amphibians—half spirit and half animal. . . . As spirits they belong to the eternal world, but as animals they inhabit time. This means that while their spirit can be directed to an eternal object, their bodies, passions, and imaginations are in continual change, for to be in time, means to change. Their nearest approach to constancy, therefore, is undulation—the repeated return to a level from which they repeatedly fall back, a series of troughs and peaks.
>
> C. S. Lewis, *The Screwtape Letters*

He is a nasty grump. A greedy, penny-pinching, crotchety character with a heart as cold as ice and as hard as steel. Ebenezer Scrooge spews bitter venom on anyone who is near. He knows he is a social pariah, but he doesn't care. In fact, it pleases him to "edge his way along the crowded paths of life, warning all human sympathy to keep its distance."[1]

We can all agree that Scrooge, whom we have either read about or seen on film in the classic *A Christmas Carol*, is a bad man, a monster even. So it is quite astonishing when, through a series of visitations from ghosts, including a tormented former business partner, he experiences an epiphany. Viewing his tragic and lonely childhood, his present contemptible existence, and his future death creates in Scrooge an impetus to change. Toward the end of the tale, a remarkable transformation takes place. Bounding from monster to humanitarian, caustic to joyful, miserly to charitable, Scrooge embodies the miraculous.

What happened to Scrooge? Was he given a new personality that Christmas Eve? No. I believe the true miracle that day was that he rediscovered who he really was. In fact, the visit from the ghost of Christmas past revealed that his goodwill and compassion had been quashed by his neglectful and cruel childhood, his mother's absence, his lack of friends at boarding school, and ultimately the loss of his only love, his exquisite fiancée, Belle. In a profoundly moving scene, she gently explains why she must leave him. "You fear the world too much. . . . All your other hopes have merged into the hope of being beyond the chance of its sordid reproach. I have seen your nobler aspirations fall off one by one, until the master-passion, Gain, engrosses you. Have I not?"[2] Clearly, there were two very different men within Scrooge, but the one overwhelmed by fear and pain buried the caring, kind, and generous one and allowed the monster to emerge.

The idea that there are two competing systems of thinking within the human brain has been well documented throughout human history. Paul, the writer of much of the New Testament and an influential leader of the early Christian church, clearly articulated the two opposing factions that constantly competed for his own mind. He wrote:

> What I don't understand about myself is that I decide one way, but then I act another, doing things I absolutely despise. . . . I realize that I don't have what it takes. I can will it, but I can't *do* it. I decide to do good, but I don't *really* do it; I decide not to do bad, but then I do it anyway. My decisions, such as they are, don't result in actions. Something has gone wrong deep within me and gets the better of me every time. (Rom. 7:15, 18–20 Message)

I sense in these words that Paul is absolutely beside himself. He feels that he is going mad. He hears proverbial voices telling him to do things that he knows will have bad outcomes, and yet he does them anyway. Paul is in the midst of a civil war in his mind. We, too, desperately desire to reconcile the warring parts of our minds to find our true selves, peace, and freedom. We want to be more patient and not overreact, but our anger gets the best of us. We want loving and peaceful marriages but continue to fight and compete with our spouses over seemingly insignificant issues. We want a good life but continue to get stuck in unhealthy or destructive cycles and relationships.

All of us have these conflicting voices shouting in our brains. So how do we make sense of a brain in constant struggle? Why do our brains work like this? Will we ever find peace?

To begin to address these vital questions, this chapter provides fundamental information about how your brain

19

works. My goal here is to describe a practical model of the human brain so you can begin to make sense of your reality. Once you do that, you can then begin to reflect on your past and recognize patterns of behaviors and emotions that have worked and those that have been destructive.

Free or Not Free?

Psychologists, philosophers, and theologians have long been fascinated by how we know ourselves, the limits of self-awareness, and the impact of not knowing ourselves. Most of us take for granted that we have free will, a choice in how we act in any situation.

It may surprise you that many biologists, psychologists, and philosophers called *determinists* or *behaviorists* believe that we have little, if any, free will. According to these camps, genes in our DNA and our early life experiences form our brain architecture, circuits, and wiring, as well as levels of nerve signals (neurotransmitters) and their receptors. Together, these genetic and physiological factors pre-program our brains in a manner that completely dictates our reactions and the thoughts that define our positions and responses to the issues we face each day. Consequently, we have little, if any, freedom in the way we act.

Determinists believe that we do not have free conscious thoughts or the ability to reason, second-guess, weigh decisions, or exert executive control over our behavioral responses. Accordingly, we lack self-control over our primal instincts because there is no self and thus no self-directed authority. For instance, a child who witnesses parental violence and repeats that same aggression had no other choice and is not responsible for their actions. Their current aggression is an inevitable outcome of the prior events experienced as a child.[3]

While there is much truth that genes and past experiences highly influence our present and future feelings, beliefs, and behaviors, is that all there is to life? What is the point of life if everything is already predetermined?

For me, one of the most troubling aspects of determinism is that good and evil, right and wrong, have no meaning. When we are simply reduced to a deterministic set of physical and chemical events, nothing is good or evil; it just is. People act how they were programmed. If this is reality, we cannot hold anyone responsible for events that had no other possible outcomes. I do not think it is an accident that the most horrible and deadly dictators of the past hundred years (such as Hitler, Stalin, Pol Pot, and Mao) all based much of their regimes' activities on deterministic philosophies. If free will and the choice between good and evil are eliminated, all that is left is humanity's capacity to destroy the weak.

In contrast to determinism, I have been influenced by the work of humanistic philosophers such as psychoanalyst Erich Fromm, particularly his books *Escape from Freedom* and *The Art of Loving*. Fromm argues that all humans have the capacity, the freedom, to change and direct their own lives; many, however, are simply too afraid to do so. This philosophical position provides a central theme found throughout this book.

I, however, like my deterministic colleagues, believe that most of us are paralyzed by the fears and primitive survival instincts from our genes, our past trauma, and a manipulative culture that constantly tries to scare us. In this state of mind, we indeed have very little free will. But unlike many determinists, I also believe that we can develop the capacity to think differently and overcome what Freud called unconscious, repressed fears and pain in order to change ourselves. This is true freedom—and freedom is the ultimate goal of our journey together.

Dual Process Reasoning (DPR)

The primary focus of this chapter, and the basis of this book, is a mind theory known as dual process reasoning (DPR). Understanding this concept is crucial for you to make sense of your reality, your behaviors, your emotions, and your thoughts.

DPR has received a great deal of attention in both the psychological and the neuroscience worlds because it provides a practical framework to describe our actions and feelings from both a physiological and a behavioral perspective. Because it offers a logical approach to discussing issues concerning the dual nature of humankind—free will and ethical responsibility—it has also gained considerable interest in philosophical and theological circles. Most recently, it has even begun to appear in sales and marketing literature as a model for designing the most effective strategies to get people to buy things.

The central idea of DPR is that there are two very distinct types of responses and reasoning that arose at distinct points during human development and that they operate in very different ways. The interaction between these two systems determines our personalities, our outlooks, our characters, our emotions, and our behaviors.

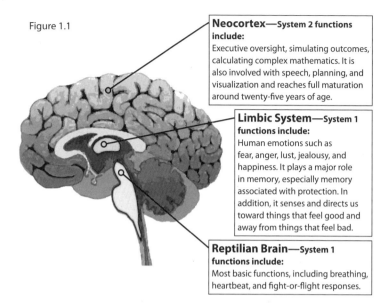

Figure 1.1

Neocortex—System 2 functions include:
Executive oversight, simulating outcomes, calculating complex mathematics. It is also involved with speech, planning, and visualization and reaches full maturation around twenty-five years of age.

Limbic System—System 1 functions include:
Human emotions such as fear, anger, lust, jealousy, and happiness. It plays a major role in memory, especially memory associated with protection. In addition, it senses and directs us toward things that feel good and away from things that feel bad.

Reptilian Brain—System 1 functions include:
Most basic functions, including breathing, heartbeat, and fight-or-flight responses.

You may have heard this theory introduced under different names (slow thinking vs. fast thinking, the unconscious vs. the conscious, reasoning vs. intuition, automatic thinking vs. controlled thinking). For the purposes of this book, I will use the terms *System 1* and *System 2*. Understanding these two systems and wiring or rewiring them in specific ways will lead you to a free and meaningful life.

It is important at this point to note my distinction between the brain and the mind. While I use both terms throughout this book and they are clearly related, there are critical differences. For me, the brain is easy to define. It is the organ of soft nervous tissue where nerve cells (neurons) communicate with the world and our bodies and control functions, movements, sensations, reasoning, feelings, and thoughts.

The mind is more mystical and complex because while it involves many of the components mentioned in regard to the brain, such as thinking, reasoning, and feeling, it combines all of these functions with the more metaphysical concept of who we are, or what I will refer to in this book (and explain more thoroughly in a bit) as the *Self*. I have illustrated the brain locations where the activities of these systems reside in Figure 1.1.

System 1

Developed over millions of years, System 1 responses are primitive reactions, feelings, sensations, and intuitions associated with animal-like survival instincts. System 1 originates predominantly from regions of the lower (reptilian) and mid (limbic system) brain and is responsible for unconscious emotions and reactions that center on survival instincts, including reproduction, protection, control, competition, and pleasure.

System 1 analysis and responses are fast, automatic, and effortless. What we see, hear, smell, taste, and touch become electrical signals that travel through the primitive portions of our brains and trigger emotions, impressions, and intuitions. We have little sense of what System 1 says to us because it is activated rapidly, without our even knowing it. Consequently, we do not have the freedom to decline or edit its messages. System 1 signals flood our brains constantly, and we can do nothing to stop them.

From a survival perspective, System 1 is highly efficient at remembering past events and particularly trauma that threatened or harmed us and unconsciously making us aware of them using fear, or flight-or-fight, responses. For example, if you are a woman and your father neglected or abandoned you when you were a child, there is a high likelihood that the threat to your well-being as a child will be transferred into adulthood as unconscious feelings of a fear of abandonment or feeling unlovable in intimate relationships. This in turn often leads to a world of heartbreak for you and others around you. These types of early cause-effect scenarios will be a central theme of this book.

Because System 1 is always on, it is responsible for much of our spontaneity as well as key aspects of social popularity and creativity. It also unconsciously performs our most familiar and practiced routines, including walking, driving, and language recognition.

System 1 plays a crucial role in one of the most basic human instincts and deeply rooted characteristics found throughout nature: survival of the fittest. For early humans, this meant the capacity to survive and eventually reproduce to pass their genes down to the next generation. In order to do this, a person had to have power to control their environment and others in that environment.

This primitive need to control is the basis of both beneficial and destructive competition evident in all aspects of the modern world. The fittest of today are individuals who successfully accumulate material possessions, rack up professional accomplishments, score sexual conquests, and increase social or wealth status, as well as those who disguise greed as ambition and dominate others in relationships.

System 2

System 2 reasoning resides in the outer regions of our brains (the neocortex and particularly the frontal cortex).

Compared to System 1 and from a neuroscience perspective, it is more sophisticated and seems to have developed very recently, only within the last one hundred fifty thousand years. Responsible for conscious thought and reasoning, it is logical and deliberate. In contrast to System 1, we know what System 2 says to us and can control when we engage this thinking.

The capacity to use System 2 to make conscious choices appears to have been a critical milestone in human history. It shifted us from being humans largely driven by our primitive, animal instincts to humans with the faculty to carry out higher-level cognitive functions, have distinct personalities, and make complex decisions.

System 2 can also monitor and intervene in certain high-stakes situations to anticipate and recognize System 1 alarms and respond in healthier and morally meaningful ways. For example, our instinctive System 1 response to a physical threat or harm by another might be to defend ourselves by hurting that person, thereby immediately eliminating the threat. However, if a teenager attempts to physically assault an adult, the adult may engage System 2 reasoning if he knows the teen and the fact that he was horribly abused growing up. Given the adult's System 2 awareness of the teenager's background, he can engage his System 2 to override System 1. He can make a reasoned choice to try not to hurt the kid. Instead, he can block the blows and hold the teenager at bay. The adult's System 2 understands the deep sense of pain experienced by the young person and reacts with grace and love, not retaliation and force.

For the purposes of this book, System 2 has five critical functions. It

1. houses the essence of who we really are;
2. reflects on complex problems and issues, weighs the pros and cons of past decisions and future options, and arrives at creative and positive solutions;
3. corrects or overrides System 1 responses when it is convinced that those responses are not beneficial to us and are harmful to others;
4. searches for and recognizes higher-level morality and the capacity to love and give selflessly; and
5. reflects God's image and allows us to intimately commune with and be in relationship with him.

I believe that the extraordinarily sophisticated neocortical brain regions that house System 2 are also where the core of who we are resides. I call this the true *Self*, a term I will henceforth capitalize and italicize throughout this book. My hope in doing so is that this typographical treatment will remind you, the reader (as well as me, the author!), of the particular meaning I intend.

Your *Self* is your individual life force that longs to be free and expressed. It makes you aware that you are a separate entity, apart from others, yet still connected to and a member of humanity. With it, you sense that from the day you were born you were a unique being, unlike anyone else on this planet.

Your *Self* encompasses the essence of who you are and who you have the potential to be. It is that part of you that gives you the capacity to balance System 1 and System 2 in a healthy and beautiful manner. Importantly, your *Self* makes it possible for you to interact with God and act in ways that reflect his image.

Your *Self* is also the part of System 2 that is capable of *Self*-reflection. In its highest form, your *Self* is a co-creator with God, because as your *Self* thinks spiritual, loving, and compassionate thoughts, those very thoughts directly form the patterns and connections within your brain circuitry that lead to loving and meaningful actions.

Your *Self* determines when it is necessary to involve other System 2 analysis and reasoning functions to balance your life and move in a healthier direction. Your *Self* can override your natural tendency to control your current situation, regret past decisions, or worry about the future. It can accept imperfections and mistakes as important learning experiences and embrace uncertainty of the future as a beautiful adventure. It gives you the capability to make free choices, which can include higher-level morality decisions and the capacity to love others without expecting anything in return. It is the intermediary and arbitrator between your eternal spirit and your animal nature, the part of your mind where you can find and experience faith.

The underpinning of this book is that although most of us have the freedom to change and the capacity to find and express our true *Selves*, we are simply too afraid or overwhelmed by our unconscious minds (reflected by System 1 responses) to do so. But the promise is that change is possible. Your true *Self*, the best you, can emerge with time, practice, and patience.

The Connection between the Two Systems

It is crucial to point out that System 1 and System 2 communicate with each other continuously via complex sets of nerve circuits or wires. Interactions between the two systems are the basis for our thoughts, actions, and personalities. Perhaps most interesting and important, especially in the context of this book, is that circuits between different brain regions can be changed or rewired by experiences and our own new thoughts and ideas. This in turn alters our behavioral habits and responses to our surroundings and the way we live. This process, known as *neuroplasticity*, is one of the most significant areas of study in neuroscience, and I will discuss it in great detail in chapter 4.

A key principle that we will come back to over and over in this book is that the more powerful an experience, habit, or thought, the stronger a brain circuit will be. The more this circuit is used, the stronger it becomes and the larger it grows. In contrast, unused brain circuits and the thoughts, behaviors, and emotions they produce weaken. Thus, what areas of life we focus on is critically important to who we become.

System 1 is a powerful force. It provides a constant and often overwhelming stream of unconscious signals. Because its functions cannot be turned off, it typically prevails over System 2's logical and conscious thoughts.

Theoretically, System 2 provides executive control over System 1. However, this requires great effort and discipline and the use of approaches such as deep *Self*-reflection, meditation, group or individual counseling, and prayer. Without regular practice of these important disciplines, the two systems operate more independently of each other and often work at cross-purposes.

Balance Matters

I want to emphasize an archetype universal in every field of science and every aspect of our lives: balance is critical. As a scientist whose work addresses processes that weaken or

Figure 1.2

System 1 Brain	System 2 Brain
Located in more primitive portions of the brain ("reptilian" brain and limbic system)	Located in the advanced portions of the brain (front brain, neocortex, and particularly the frontal cortex)
Acts fast and effortlessly	Acts slowly and requires effort to get involved
Houses the unconscious *Self*	Houses the conscious *Self*
Recognizes and responds to danger with fear and action; remembers previously experienced threats	Calculates and simulates outcomes after weighing the pros and cons of a situation
Drives survival and competitive instincts	Critical for higher level morality and sacrificial choices
Triggers emotions (intuitions, impressions, desire, and feelings)	Responsible for deliberative, logical, and deductive reasoning, including mathematical statistics
Responsible for impulses, habits, drives, and reactions that give rise to creativity and spontaneity	Creates and analyzes abstract concepts
Looks for immediate causes and patterns, especially those that resemble past events	Reflects in consideration of bigger picture options
Often inaccurate and is incapable of fact-checking	Capable of fact-checking and executive function to override System 1 reactions and responses

sicken the human body, I can tell you that balance matters. If one biological system is out of control while another designed to control or counter that original system is diminished, our bodies will not work properly and typically will damage themselves.

System 1 is not bad and System 2 good, or vice versa. We need them both to live healthy lives. When one system is in constant overdrive, the other underfunctions and we feel and behave in ways that dramatically limit our capacity to experience joy. Therefore, the two systems must be balanced. Figure 1.2 gives a summary of the specific characteristics of the two systems.

System 1 has a number of key advantages, including helping us rapidly respond to a crisis or danger and perform daily tasks like walking and driving. It is also responsible for much of our spontaneity, creativity, and intuition. Let's also be clear. Feelings, sensations, and responses from System 1 can be fun and quite pleasurable (some of which will be explored in chapter 10).

But what it means to be human involves System 2. Its functions help us understand we are unique entities with the incredible capacity to *Self*-reflect. We can make free choices, look at the big picture, and simulate a wide range of outcomes. System 2 also allows us to make selfless choices and connect with our Creator.

So we need them both, in *balance*.

I have seen System 1 compared to Homer on the hit TV show *The Simpsons* and System 2 to Spock on *Star Trek* or Data on *Star Trek: The Next Generation* (depending on your age). While this may not be the most scientific analogy, it does allow us to think about the different capabilities and the advantages and disadvantages of the two systems.

Take Homer, for instance. He's a fun guy, the life of the party, unpredictable. While he would probably be a blast to hang out with for an evening, Homer would also most likely act irrationally in the face of danger and make impulsive decisions without considering others.

Now think about Spock and Data. While not the most creative, spontaneous, or fun-loving types, these guys would help you analyze and solve a complex problem. They would likely remain calm in a stressful situation and do what they thought was right without emotional input.

While these three characters have great qualities in their own right, wouldn't it be great if we could balance them out? Luckily for us, I believe we can beautifully balance the spontaneous, fun-loving, creative, and social aspects of System 1 with System 2's capacity for deep introspective analysis, sophisticated problem solving, and higher-level morality. Think Captain James T. Kirk, Captain Jean-Luc Picard, and Marge.

In his book *Strangers to Ourselves*, Timothy Wilson points out that most mundane tasks of living are delegated to the unconscious mind. The conscious mind, System 2, is like the CEO of a large company, and the employees who carry out the daily activities are like the unconscious mind, System 1. The beautiful and delicate balance of roles between CEO and employees is what makes a company (life) successful.[4]

A company will go awry if the CEO or its employees do not do their jobs or misuse or neglect their positions and power. For example, if the CEO does not know everyone's roles, fails to focus and direct the company, or neglects the executive role of vision, oversight, and correction, the company will fail. The CEO must constantly monitor the organization, know their *Self*, and understand the purpose of the company. When they do so, all components of the organization are efficient and work well together to move it in the right direction.

If, however, the employees rally, take over the company, and move it in an unhealthy and destructive direction without the CEO's intervention, the company will deteriorate into chaos and devastation.

This can be true in our lives. If System 1 runs rampant without System 2 oversight, we can suffer in cycles of broken relationships, sadness, depression, unhealthy obsessions, and overwhelming fear. It is up to us to find our *Selves* within

System 2 to direct System 1 to turn the ship around and stop destructive behaviors.

A Downward Spiral

It does not matter how small the sins are provided that their cumulative effect is to edge the man away from the Light and out into the Nothing. Murder is no better than cards if cards can do the trick. Indeed the safest road to Hell is the gradual one—the gentle slope, soft underfoot, without sudden turnings, without milestones, without signposts.[5]

We humans have an incredible capacity to adapt to whatever path we are on, no matter how dysfunctional or unmanageable. Ironically, unless we learn *Self*-reflection to monitor our pain, we will remain stuck in the same recurring situations, never considering that we might need to change.

C. S. Lewis is my favorite author and greatest contemporary influence. One of his most popular books, *The Screwtape Letters*, is a series of thirty-one letters from Screwtape, a senior demon, to his nephew Wormwood, a junior tempter who is trying to get a man into hell.

In the above quotation, the senior demon reminds his nephew that it is best not to lure the man toward the "big" sins (like murder and adultery) because a life absent of *Self*-examination, reflection, and honesty will do the trick and carry less risk. It is much safer to let the man think that while his life might not be ideal, it is better than most and there is no need to change course. In other words, keep it simple.

Keep the man's pain at a tolerable level, and he will not wake up. Assure him he is a decent fellow, but at the same time encourage him to repeat the same mistakes and the same negative behavioral patterns. Keep him stuck in the same toxic relationship cycles with his wife, family, and friends. And never, ever allow the man to consider for one moment that his troubles may be of his own making. No, no, no. Settle in the man's mind that his problems are his wife's, his friends', his neighbors', his co-workers', and his mother's fault. Then your job is done, and your man safely makes it to hell.

Does this scare you as much as it scares me? As I reflect on my life, I was, many times, on that gradual downward slope, falling deeper and deeper into the throes of pain and loneliness (more on this in the next chapter). I was walking around in a make-believe dream world, never aware of the true reality around me. Perhaps most frightening was that at the time I was convinced that I was just fine.

Oh, I knew I was unhealthy. I had high blood pressure and was diagnosed with depression and was regularly seeing doctors to treat these conditions with medication.

At the time, I believed these illnesses resulted from a combination of my genetics and a chemical imbalance that could be treated with prescriptive meds. Today, however, I believe that my System 1 overreaction responses were the basis of most of my emotional and physical pain.

Our minds and our bodies cannot endure constant and overwhelming feelings such as fear, anger, pain, regret, and resentment that come into our lives each day without serious physical and emotional repercussions. Eventually, we break. Our minds and bodies get sick. We don't know why we are falling apart because these feelings arise from the unconscious mind (System 1), which is inaccessible to us. Consequently, we cannot consciously process and make sense of them. All we know is that we hurt badly and are deeply depressed and incredibly lonely.

The United States claims the highest rates of mental illness in the world. More than 25 percent of Americans report they suffer from mental illness; the most common are anxiety and mood disorders.[6] Research also estimates that more than half of Americans will experience mental illness during their lifetimes.[7] These diseases devastate our society; incapacitate our personal, social, and work lives; cost the United States over three hundred billion dollars and more each year; and cause premature death.[8] I believe that System 1 in overdrive is much of the basis of our mental illnesses. In the next chapter, you are going to learn why that is.

Modern society makes it easy to numb our pain rather than address the problem. Our unhealthy compulsions, addictive tendencies, depression, and mood disorders can be dulled just enough to prevent our pain from reaching a level that awakens us to our need to change.

Don't get me wrong. I value the external healing powers of integrative medicine, prescription medications, and cognitive and psychodynamic therapies. I am fully aware that oftentimes medications help people function and stay alive. That said, I advocate that we need a new language and approach to teach individuals how to balance System 1 and 2 responses so they can optimize their strengths as opposed to only treating symptoms.

So how do we find and fix the problem? It starts with learning to think and do differently.

I am reminded of my pole-vaulting experience in college. During many a track team practice, after my numerous failed attempts to clear the bar, my coach would scream, "Ski, you are not getting high enough!" I was always tempted to respond, "No kidding, Captain Obvious." My coach never understood that yelling was not an effective means to help me change my approach. I needed instructions on what I could do differently to correct the part of my jump that needed to be fixed.

Likewise, it is useless to keep telling someone:

"Snap out of it!"
"Work harder. Try again!"
"Stop being so obsessive (or controlling or sad or anxious)!"
"Just say no to drugs, alcohol, promiscuity, or binge eating!"

You need to understand the source(s) of your problems, fears, and pain and equip your *Self* with the tools and approaches that will help you move up and over the bar to your goals, far away from the downward slope. We aim to help you do this throughout this book.

This Works!

Understanding dual process reasoning has been the most important discovery of my life. It has allowed me to make sense of my current reality, change my past damaging behaviors, and find and express my true *Self*.

I use this model practically every day to analyze situations and take a more reasoned, conscious approach to resolving them. I say things like, "Ski, you are acting very System 1 in this circumstance. Is that really how you want to look at this problem? Is there truly a threat that you should be responding to like that?" Or when interacting with another, I will often think, "That person desperately needs control.

I don't believe it is safe to work with them or that I would enjoy working with them." While I was writing this book, my twenty-nine-year-old son and his friends picked up the lingo. Now I overhear them say, "Man, I'm System 1-ing out today. This girl (or situation) has me freaked out!"

With use of the dual process reasoning approach, I am free to give my feelings and reactions a name and understand where they come from. I am free to shift when I judge others with negative adjectives such as "mean," "selfish," and "bad" and instead recognize the imbalance in the two systems of thinking. I am also free to understand when I can't influence another's behavior and must therefore put boundaries in place. Now I can focus on what I can change: my thoughts and how I choose to act.

That said, I am not perfect. I have a deep System 1 drive that believes I can fix any situation, any person, anything. My default thoughts sometimes scream, "Look at me! I went from a house without a bathroom in rural North Carolina to being rapidly promoted through the academic ranks at Johns Hopkins and Wake Forest. I can remedy anything, and with enough effort, I can't be stopped!" Unfortunately, my hard work to change the opinions or behaviors of others has gotten me into a world of trouble. I will talk about the reason for this System 1 drive in chapter 2, but for now let's just say that Melody Beattie's *Codependent No More* lives on the nightstand next to my bed.

Reflection: The Pathway to Rewire Your Mind

The first step to rewire your brain is to realize something is wrong in your life. While you do not have to identify exactly

what that is just yet, take some time to pause and answer the
questions below. These are designed to help you begin the
process of *Self*-reflection and discovery.

1. Do you have overwhelming feelings and emotions in
   your mind concerning important areas of your life?
   What are they?
2. Have you faced difficult or even devastating situations
   and question how you handled them? Choose one and
   think about what you could have done differently.
3. Are there times when, like the apostle Paul, you know
   the right thing to do but do the opposite? Why do you
   think that is?
4. Do you believe your future is predetermined and you
   have little or no power to change it? Why or why not?

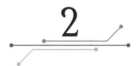

2

Stuck in Overdrive

> I've got 99 problems and 86 of them are completely made up scenarios in my head that I'm stressing about for absolutely no logical reason.
>
> Unknown

I have an incredible fear that has been difficult for me to overcome. I am claustrophobic. This phobia is particularly difficult to deal with when I am on an airplane, and I do a lot of air travel. Although anxiety begins to build when the aircraft door shuts, as long as everything proceeds in an expected manner, I can deal with it. However, if there is a delay in any part of the process of getting into the air or getting to the gate after touching down, I develop a paralyzing fear almost to the point of believing I will go crazy. My chest tightens. My heart rate increases. My breaths become short and rapid. There are times I am right on the edge of my seat ready to shout, "If I don't get off this airplane, I'm going to die!"

Consciously, I realize these thoughts are completely irrational. Do you know anyone who has ever been stuck on an airplane for days, months, or years? Or do you know anyone, outside of victims of rare crashes, who has died on an airplane? I am absolutely aware that my fear is out of proportion, but that does not make my panic any less real.

The other night while I was working on this chapter, this fear reemerged. I had flown from Los Angeles to Cincinnati, where I boarded a connecting flight to Charlotte. I won't mention names of any airlines, but this particular night three planes destined for Charlotte failed their safety checks. By the time I crawled onto the third one, it was midnight and the temperature had fallen below zero. The plane moved out onto the runway and then pulled over to the side. It sat there for over an hour without any information from the pilot. Within the first fifteen minutes, anxiety set in. *Why aren't we moving? Has the plane's engine or hydraulics failed due to the temperature? Are we going to stay in this small plane in Cincinnati all night? Does anyone even know we're here? I've got to get off this plane! Do I fake a heart attack?*

God really does have a sense of humor. I believe this was his way of using one of my greatest, and on the surface most irrational, fears to keep the content of this chapter real. The suffocating feelings I have on an airplane make it seem like my warning system is absurd and not working properly. But in the moment, the suffocating feelings and sensations I have on an airplane tell me I am in great danger. The intensity of this System 1, unconscious reaction increases with every passing minute of a delay. The escalating fear and anxiety eventually result in a powerful drive to get off the plane.

Over the years, I have worked hard through extensive counseling to reflect on my fear. Where does it come from? Why does it appear? I believe it is impossible in many cases to know the exact nexus of such a fear, but based on my *Self*-exploration, I believe in my case two childhood events are prime candidates.

One, as a child, I was the victim of bullying by some older boys. Every time my family made its weekly Sunday trip to the local swimming pool, these kids got their kicks by holding me under the water, often until I passed out. Two, I was sexually assaulted as a child by a family acquaintance for several months. This individual held me down as he abused me. In both cases, someone stronger and bigger overpowered and hurt me.

I believe these early events created a heightened and desperate need to be in control of my personal space. When I am not, especially if I am confined in a closed area, I feel the same panic I felt when I was being bullied and abused and subsequently transfer that emotion onto my current situation. As it turns out, I am not alone. A large body of science has documented how exposure to trauma such as childhood bullying or abuse can have a lasting psychological impact on a person as an adult.[1]

System 1 responses such as the ones I experienced may have been legitimate and necessary for survival in an initial experience. However, as time passes and we move from our traumatic childhood experience(s) to adulthood, the automatic reactions we endure (such as my fight-or-flight response on airplanes) no longer serve a useful purpose. In fact, such

System 1 dysfunctions only cause pain, discomfort, and/or obsessions that can make our lives miserable and at times completely unmanageable.

I believe that most of us living in modern societies suffer from a profound imbalance between System 1 and System 2 emotions and behaviors. This leaves many of us in perpetual fear and anxiety, with a need to control, and suffering from obsessions, compulsions, habits, dependencies, and addictions.

Inaccurate by Nature

Perhaps the primary weakness of System 1 is that it is often not accurate. On autopilot, it does not calculate the likelihood of potential outcomes and risks. In his book *Thinking, Fast and Slow*, Daniel Kahneman focuses on the prevalence of human thinking errors in our society. This work is an extensive examination of the biases of our fast-thinking System 1 and how we incorrectly and automatically believe that our feelings and intuitions are much more accurate than they actually are.[2]

System 1 is fast, much faster than System 2. It does not have the capacity to fact-check information. Since System 2 cannot easily recognize System 1 activity (because it happens without our knowing it), System 2 typically cannot confirm the System 1–induced responses. Consequently, System 1 produces fears, impulses, judgments, and reactions to stimuli and events with no ability to assess actual risk. While it does a great job detecting the potential of a hazard and identifying the reactions needed to evade the danger, System 1 lacks the capacity to validate that the perceived threat was really dangerous.

In his book *Strangers to Ourselves*, Timothy Wilson offers an illustration of this System 1 deficit. If you spot a menacing-looking snake while walking a trail in the woods, your System 1 will quickly produce great fear, particularly if you are afraid of snakes. It will automatically turn on your fight-or-flight response to move you immediately in another direction to find safety. However, because System 1 does not fact-check, its immediate deduction may not be accurate. For example, maybe what looks like a snake is really just a stick or maybe a harmless black snake that kills poisonous snakes.[3]

System 2 needs to be activated in order for you to further assess the details of a situation and make these determinations. However, most people who are afraid of snakes will not stick around to look into other possibilities. On the contrary, they will run as fast as possible out of the woods, thinking and telling anyone who will listen that they just eluded death after coming face-to-face with a venomous rattlesnake the size of their arm. Insidiously, such an event can shake their psyche for weeks, months, and even years. If their fear of snakes is great enough, they may never again enter the woods. All of this takes place because of a stick in the middle of a trail that looked like a snake.

This is what System 1 in overdrive has the capacity to do to us. Many of us overreact to literally thousands of perceived threats daily, which leave us in a constant state of fear and suspicion. As a result, we miss out on the beauty of what is possible. These overreactive responses take enormous energy and disconnect us from positive experiences. If we never go back into the woods because we are too scared of finding another snake, we will forever miss the splendor of the forest, the autumn colors of the hardwoods, and the melodies of a song sparrow. In a similar vein, if we overestimate the risk of crime in our neighborhoods, we will spend most of our lives indoors and miss out on meeting others and playing in the fresh air with our kids. If we fear that every person sitting next to us on an airplane, bus, or subway might have Ebola or be a terrorist, we will refuse to travel and will never see beautiful parts of our country and the world.

Competition

Another aspect of an elevated System 1 response that can be particularly destructive is an excessive survival of the fittest or competition instinct. I am going to talk about this in depth in several of the chapters in this book, but it is important to mention it here as it can produce significant and damaging results when in overdrive.

At its best, competition serves a vital function to improve societies. It drives performance, quality, choice, economic development, and innovation to make us better in many areas of life. We Americans, in particular, love and even thrive in the face of this strong natural instinct.

Competition centers on the power and capacity to control someone or something and come out on top. If one sports team is stronger or faster or has a better coach than another, it wins. If one company has a competitive advantage (innovation, supply chain, marketing) over another, it wins.

While these are generally harmless examples, competition can weave destruction. For instance, conflicts between individuals in families and intimate relationships, racial groups, nations, and religions can be devastating on both a personal and a far-reaching, even global, level.

At the heart of most human violence sits our primal instinct to control what we perceive puts us at risk in our environment. When humans encounter a person or a group of people who are different (whether in gender, race, religion, political affiliation, sexual orientation, or nationality), System 1 and its primitive origins kick in. It automatically sends out unconscious signals (intuitions and feelings) that the individual or group is a potential threat. And unless we allow System 2 to intervene, things can get ugly quickly. Just see what happens when two aggressive species of animals occupy the same cage and compete for the same food.

In his landmark book *The Seat of the Soul*, Gary Zukav writes,

> The same energy that separated the family of Romeo from the family of Juliet is the same energy that separates the racial family of the black husband from the racial family of the white wife. The same energy that set Lee Harvey Oswald against John F. Kennedy is the same energy that set Cain against Abel. Brothers and sisters quarrel for the same reason corporations quarrel—they seek power over one another.[4]

This is why the nonviolent protests of individuals such as Martin Luther King Jr. and Mahatma Gandhi are so extraordinary. I recently watched the movie *Selma*, which documents the true story of King's fight to secure equal voting rights in Alabama in 1965. I was reminded of the incredible System 2 courage and choice that this iconic civil rights activist exhibited while peaceably marching into crowds full of people brandishing weapons, hurling racial slurs, and even using physical force. In contrast, our System 1 tendency is to fight back and create more chaos, confusion, and violence. I believe

King's nonviolent System 2 approach is the only way the fabric of a racially divided nation can be changed for the better.

A key principle of competition is who has the power. Power can be taken, given, bought, stolen, or inherited from someone or something. It is essential to remember that when power is transferred from one entity to another, one's gain will come at the expense of another's loss. When all the wealth in a country is concentrated within the hands of a few, it is shifted from the majority. When one person in a relationship dominates the other, power shifts from the dominated to the dominator. The moment a healthy individual begins to feel controlled or overpowered in a relationship is the moment that intimacy begins to dissipate.

We were all born with the System 1 instinct to compete and control our environments for *Self*-preservation. But we must learn how to recognize and understand when survival instincts are appropriate and beneficial and when they are destructive and detrimental. *Self*-awareness and *Self*-control, not the control of others, build the human capacity to connect, cooperate, and create and maintain harmonious lives and relationships. Such actions require a deep understanding of the *Self* and seemingly paradoxical System 2 choices like those Christ expressed in the Beatitudes. I love the way Eugene Peterson articulates these blessings in his paraphrase *The Message*.

> You're blessed when you're content with just who you are—no more, no less. That's the moment you find yourselves proud owners of everything that can't be bought.
>
> You're blessed when you've worked up a good appetite for God. He's food and drink in the best meal you'll ever eat.
>
> You're blessed when you care. At the moment of being "care-full," you find yourselves cared for.

You're blessed when you get your inside world—your mind and heart—put right. Then you can see God in the outside world.

You're blessed when you can show people how to cooperate instead of compete or fight. That's when you discover who you really are, and your place in God's family. (Matt. 5:5–9)

These are beautiful and poignant words, reminders of what is possible when we recognize and refuse to live under the rule of System 1 in overdrive. Though we may long to be, not many of us are in that place.

The Undifferentiated Individual

I describe people who approach most situations in life with System 1 in overdrive as *undifferentiated*, a term I will use throughout this book. I want to assure you that I associate no judgment with this word. Many people who operate with dominant System 1 emotions and behaviors experienced earlier (perhaps childhood) trauma in their lives that has driven their feelings and responses.

The term *differentiation* is often used in biology and medicine and sometimes in psychology to describe how well an entity, whether an individual cell or a person, has become specialized or matured toward its ultimate purpose. Embryonic stem cells, for instance, are undifferentiated. Depending on the environment to which they are exposed, they can differentiate, or develop and mature, into more than two hundred cell types that make up the human body.[5]

Now the downside to undifferentiated cells. A key event that leads to many cancers is when a particular cell type within a tissue is transformed from differentiated to undifferentiated.

When this change occurs, all hell breaks loose because the undifferentiated cells can replicate much more rapidly than adjacent differentiated cells, and they also refuse to die after a certain period of time. When a group of undifferentiated cells within an organ like the liver can proliferate out of control and not perish, they rapidly take over the liver as a cancer and eventually kill the person if not treated.

I believe this is analogous to undifferentiated people driven by System 1 fears and responses that limit their abilities to manage emotions and develop healthy relationships. Fear and paranoia responses escalate, isolate, and disconnect individuals to the point that it is difficult for them to mature enough to enjoy or find purpose in life. System 1 in overdrive also can lead to destructive behaviors and responses that affect people around them and especially loved ones. Undifferentiated people are imprisoned by an overactive System 1 and do not even know it. They are convinced they are right and the world is wrong.

The Prison We Find Ourselves In

Most people believe they orchestrate their own lives. They are convinced they make and follow their own ideas and inclinations. For most of us most of the time, however, this is simply not true. While I have already talked about things like unruly emotions, control issues, and unmanageable situations, these are not our prisons. I like to think of them as our jailors.

The prison is found in the organization of our brains that generates the overactivity of System 1. The primary reason we have such difficulty knowing our *Selves* and controlling our actions is that we do not have access to most of what is happening in our brains. We are, as psychology professor Timothy Wilson points out in his book of the same title, "strangers to ourselves." This is why we have trouble directing our thoughts and actions. It is also why we often behave in ways that are destructive to our *Selves* and to others for reasons that are completely a mystery to us.

Scientists have estimated that the unconscious mind has the ability to interpret and respond to over ten thousand nerve signals per second, or about fifteen million signals per day. This is in stark contrast to the conscious mind, which is estimated to process only forty nerve signals per second (about sixty thousand per day).[6] This means that 99.6 percent of the nerve signals in our brains take place without our knowing or having access to them. Is it any wonder that we often have "99 problems and 86 of them are completely made up scenarios in my head that I'm stressing about for absolutely no logical reason"?

Many unconscious nerve signals are designed to serve our five senses, and others are critical for life-sustaining activities (such as organ function and respiration). However, our brains also produce an overwhelming number of unconscious System 1 signals that affect our feelings, emotions, and behavioral reactions without our knowing it. This is so powerful because our conscious System 2 cannot make sense of the continuous and overwhelming noise.

When System 1 is always in overdrive, we interpret the world as a place with emergencies everywhere. Most situations we encounter seem to pose a serious threat to our survival. Thus, we overreact with exaggerated System 1 responses in the most vital parts of our lives time and time

49

again. Our conscious System 2 just can't keep up. In fact, studies show that chronic stress, anxiety, depression, PTSD, and addictions all alter the metabolism, function, and even size of brain regions involved with System 2 thinking. Overwhelmed by System 1's chaos, System 2 underfunctions or shuts itself down and allows anarchy to reign. Now we are prisoners of our own minds.

My Prison

I was raised in a small farming community in rural North Carolina in the late 1960s and early 1970s. Though the children in our community regularly attended school, caring for tobacco crops and playing sports were far more important than reading, writing, and arithmetic. Consequently, neither schoolteachers nor administrators recognized or addressed learning disabilities like dyslexia.

Being severely dyslexic, though I didn't know it at the time, I struggled to read and write, especially in middle school. My teachers assumed I was mentally disabled, or, as it was commonly termed and widely accepted back then, "retarded."

Children with special needs and challenges of varying degrees (including severe developmental delay, ADHD, autism, dyslexia, and serious behavioral issues) were placed in a little white building outside the main school area. This little white building became my new home during sixth and seventh grade. The assigned teachers didn't teach us anything because they didn't know how to in light of our challenges. So for seven hours, five days a week, we kids were holed up in that little white building while teachers constantly yelled at us to "shut up." Being there for two years produced in me an incredible amount of stress and anxiety. Perhaps more notably, it destroyed my *Self*-worth.

The lack of sensitivity for basic human dignity, let alone the will to educate and nurture children who were different in that day, was clearly unacceptable. Not only was it okay to use the word *retarded*, but classrooms were also labeled in visibly discriminatory ways. For instance, the smartest kids belonged in the "A" class. The "B" class was for kids with average intelligence. The "C" class claimed the not-so-bright students. And then there was the "D" class, mine, referred to by students and teachers alike as the "retards" and often the butt of cruel jokes. Day after day, schoolmates and even some teachers made it crystal clear who and where I was—"a retarded boy in the little white building."

When I tell this story today, people always ask how I escaped the little white building. This part is actually kind of funny. The state required all students to take an IQ test at the beginning of eighth grade. I remember taking the test and thinking how easy it was. Naturally, I assumed it had been redesigned especially for our class and that my fellow classmates were enjoying the test as much as I was.

I must have done well because when the results came back, teachers lavished unusually positive attention on me and instantly transferred me to the "A" class. Unfortunately, that move created in me more insecurity because I still couldn't read or learn to read. I suspected everyone in that class was quietly thinking, "Oh, for Pete's sake. Send the poor kid back to the retarded class already."

This experience left me with lasting scars and not just of an obvious emotional or psychological nature. According to the latest data in neuroscience literature, including my own, this type of trauma also affected the very chemical nature of my DNA and how my brain circuitry formed. I discuss this in great detail in chapter 4. All of these environmental-biological interactions gave rise to specific and negative brain wiring, feelings, and, consequently, behaviors. They also occurred at a time in my life when they could do a lot of damage. Even though I was cognitively unaware of my System 1 feelings, the circuitry patterns that would cause a deep sense of rejection, abandonment, inferiority, and depression for most of my adult life were put in place at an early age.

My sister once wisely told me, "The 'retarded' class will do one of two things, Ski. It will either crush you or it will make you great." I opted for the latter. After graduating high school, I hit the ground running. I accumulated degrees. It took me only three years (versus the average of five to six) to get a PhD in biochemistry at Wake Forest University School of Medicine. I am told that I still hold the record for getting a PhD in the shortest amount of time in the history of that program. During this time, I practically lived in the laboratory and slept there most nights. In fact, on one particular Christmas, my parents threatened to call the police to commit me if I didn't leave the building that day. I was obsessed!

I made a name in the prestigious worlds of academia, science, publishing, and business. I was a very successful professor at Johns Hopkins and Wake Forest, published over one hundred thirty scientific articles and four popular diet books, held over thirty patents, and started several companies, one of which I took public as president and CEO. I worked eighteen- to twenty-hour days in an effort to make myself "worthy," the pictorial definition of success. And yet I was severely depressed and lonely, even to the point of needing to take several medications.

While preparing a press kit for one of my earlier books, my publisher asked me to write a brief biography of my life. I spent a couple of hours working on it. When I read it aloud, I experienced an epiphany.

As clear as a reflection in a mirror was the fact that my almost superhuman desire to succeed was not motivated by a joy of accomplishment but by an intense drive to be accepted, recognized, loved, and most of all not be called "retarded." No matter how successful I was, I remained a frightened little boy who would do anything to never again, metaphorically speaking, be sent back to the retarded class. Every choice I made stemmed from a deep and persistent fear seated in a primitive portion of my brain. This fear was a survival response, an unhealthy emotional reaction created and fueled by traumatic events in my childhood.

My relationships were also negatively impacted by my inferiority belief system. In order to be loved, I felt I needed to do something to deserve it. Unconsciously, I was drawn to those who needed help because I unconsciously believed they might somehow love me if I helped them. This created extremely destructive codependent issues in both of my marriages and ultimately played a huge role in their demise.

I now realize that though I had believed I was making reasoned decisions, I was not. I was simply reacting over and over with basic survival System 1 feelings and responses that were in overdrive. My emotions and behaviors were programmed so deeply in me, stemming from that little white building, that I was destined to repeat them time and time again. In fact, it took me almost forty years to realize I was in that prison and begin to escape it.

Others suffer more than I could ever imagine. I was blessed to have had loving parents who encouraged me. I know many are not so fortunate. The tragedy of living in this imperfect world is that pain and brokenness are inevitable. It is safe to assume that we will be hurt at some point in our lives. So the question is not Will we suffer? but How will we handle the damage from our most traumatic experiences? Specifically, how will we deal with the brain wiring and resulting behavioral dysfunctions that are a consequence of these experiences? The answer to the latter question will determine everything about our future.

Powerful Dysfunctions Require Powerful Change

Kimerer LaMothe says that "our emotional responses can become habits that color our reactions to things without our really knowing it."[7] I, too, believe that our consistent reactions based solely on our System 1 feelings (desire, anger, fear, anxiety, hurt, jealousy, unworthiness, inadequacy) in overdrive can lead to powerful emotional dysfunctions that have the capacity to diminish our well-being and even destroy our lives. An emotional dysfunction is a condition in which we feel an emotion or react in a way that is out of proportion to the current situation. For example, we may lose our tempers when a relatively minor goal is blocked or feel weighed down with sadness when to most eyes our lives are going well. The brain wiring for these dysfunctions typically is created as a coping mechanism to promote survival and avert pain in a difficult, if not life-threatening, situation in childhood or the adolescent years.

Clearly, my early experience of being placed in an environment that tore down my value as a human hardwired in me an emotional dysfunction, a need to guarantee by any means necessary that I was acceptable and lovable. People who suffer from low *Self*-esteem and question whether they are lovable may be dependent on others for constant attention and validation. Those who greatly fear the uncertainty of the future may be bent toward controlling their environment and others in it. We will address more dysfunctions in future chapters.

Throughout this book, Dr. Rukstalis and I will constantly remind you that you can change and now is the time. Don't wait forty years like I did to discover what has prevented your joy. However, because you have been the way you are for many years, this process will take time. Change will be gradual even under the best circumstances as you learn how to *Self*-direct the rewiring of your mind. The capacity to rewire your mind will depend on several factors, including

1. how well you understand the framework of your mind and the source of your pain,
2. the depth of your System 1 scars,
3. how much you want to change,
4. whether you have humility and can be vulnerable enough to surrender your old way of life to God, and
5. the effort and discipline you put into learning.

I am a work in progress. Thanks to intensive counseling, personal research into the philosophy and psychology of the mind, two cancer scares, painful inner excavating, a deep desire to be different, and surrendering to God my unconscious System 1 belief that I was unacceptable and unlovable, I was able to begin to transform my thinking, my behavioral patterns, and my future. My life now has great joy, meaning, and freedom.

It won't be easy, but you can find joy, meaning, and freedom too.

Reflection: The Pathway to Rewire Your Mind

1. Can you identify situations in your life when you responded in an exaggerated or illogical manner that was destructive to you or others? Perhaps you suffer from a phobia or you have a tendency to overreact emotionally. What are the situations that trigger you? How do you tend to respond?

2. Did you experience or do you suspect you experienced a traumatic event as a child? If so, how has it significantly affected your life today?

3. Have you ever considered the concept of emotional dysfunction? What does it mean to you?

4. One example of an emotional dysfunction was my need to guarantee by any means necessary that I was acceptable and lovable. Reflect on your life, your behaviors, your habits, and your reactions. Could you be suffering from an emotional dysfunction? If so, what? How is your behavior out of proportion to the current situation?

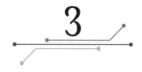

Fear-Obsessed

If we let things terrify us, then life is not worth living.

Seneca, Roman philosopher

The mood in the conference room is tense. Clouds of cigarette smoke float around the executives from the Sterling Cooper Advertising Agency and their biggest client, tobacco company Lucky Strike. As the men in sharp suits puff on their top-selling product, Roger Sterling, the head of the ad agency, gives some bad news. They are no longer able to advertise a "safer" cigarette for their client.

The meeting goes downhill from there.

The ad execs offer a few ultimately bad ideas, one by a wet-behind-the-ears junior executive that revolves around a "death wish." Exasperated, the cigarette company's top dogs end the meeting and start to walk out of the room.

After a long minute, just enough to amplify the drama, it is Don Draper to the rescue. With his dark, slicked-back hair, expensive suit, and handsome looks, he reels possibility back in with his smooth voice by saying, "Advertising is based on one thing: happiness. And do you know what happiness is? Happiness is the smell of a new car. It's freedom from fear. It's a billboard on the side of a road that screams with reassurance that whatever you're doing is okay. You are okay."[1]

These profound words, featured in a scene from the season premier of the hit show *Mad Men*, not only win the hearts of the Lucky Strike execs but also ring true today. Don Draper is right. Happiness is freedom from fear.

In conducting research for this book, I was surprised to discover that outside of philosophy, psychology, and theology, dual process reasoning (DPR) is widely discussed in the sales and marketing industry. This industry understands that System 1 reactions to fear will drive consumers to purchase products. This is why market researchers associated with advertising most major commercial products spend enormous amounts of time and money to determine our greatest fears and how to exploit them.

We are constantly bombarded with products that create or magnify and ultimately promise to remedy our anxieties, whether we fear being unattractive, having bad breath, not being a good enough parent, getting cancer, or even passing up a great deal.

Think about how easy it is for a mother to believe she needs a security system after she sees a television advertisement spotlighting two dangerous-looking men breaking into a home. Or for a twentysomething to feel like he is missing out on leading a tech-savvy and full life if he doesn't purchase the latest smartphone or Apple gadget.

Martin Lindstrom, author of *Brandwashed* and *Buyology*, says, "Some advertisers prey on our fears of our worst selves by activating insecurities we didn't even know we had."[2] Using Dove's "go sleeveless" ad campaign as an illustration, Lindstrom shows how this beauty company subconsciously made women fear not just how bad their armpits smelled but how they looked as well. He asserts this campaign was founded in advertising techniques made popular in the 1920s that "(a) pinpoint a problem, perhaps one consumers didn't even know they had; (b) exacerbate anxiety around the problem; and (c) sell the cure."[3]

Yes, fear sells. And we're buying.

The Problem of Fear

Franklin D. Roosevelt is one of my favorite presidents. I especially admire how he led the United States through numerous hardships, including the Great Depression and World War II. In his first and short 1,883-word inaugural speech on March 4, 1933, President Roosevelt stated up front what many believe to be some of the most critical words ever spoken to this country.

> So, first of all, let me assert my firm belief that the only thing we have to fear is . . . fear itself—nameless, unreasoning, unjustified terror which paralyzes needed efforts to convert retreat into advance.[4]

Why was this so important? At that time, our nation had already endured three years of a devastating depression in which almost half (eleven thousand out of twenty-four thousand) of all banks had failed, wiping out the accounts of their depositors. Millions were out of work, with millions more barely living above subsistence. The currency and farm markets had completely eroded. In the face of this enormous adversity, President Roosevelt focused his address on fear and how it, not the current situation, could destroy the country.

I do not want you to miss this: the System 1 emotion of fear typically is the most influential force that wires our brains and the biggest roadblock to rewiring and change. Fear is paralyzing because it prevents our development, our maturation into well-adapted people. It keeps us from taking meaningful actions to address our most difficult circumstances. In the face of our worst problems, powerful addictions, miserable relationships, and general unhappiness and dissatisfaction with life, fear is our biggest enemy.

Before we give this primitive emotion too much authority, know that fear has one basic job: to provide information in order to protect us. Joseph LeDoux of the Center of Fear and Anxiety at New York University said, "We come into the world knowing how to be afraid. We learn what to be afraid of."[5] Learning fear is driven by the information we are exposed to or expose ourselves to, as well as the credibility we give the source of the information regarding the threat. This is why it is necessary to activate System 2. We must use its reasoning capacity to assess the accuracy of System 1 information. We will discuss how to do so in the most critical areas of our lives in the second part of this book.

Exaggerated fear is problematic because it creates unfounded paranoia; it paralyzes us and narrows our focus, thereby blocking our capacity to change. When fear takes over, all is lost because we cannot alter the System 1 emotional dysfunctions that have made our lives a nightmare.

Fear Comes in Many Packages

When recovering addicts work through step 4 of the Alcoholics Anonymous twelve-step program, they are asked to make a moral inventory of their lives. To help guide them through the process of taking stock of their fears, *The Big Book*, on which the program is based, offers a "Fear Inventory Prompt List."[6] See if you resonate with any of these in Figure 3.1. (Note: This list is not exhaustive.)

Since fears are automatic instincts that are typically learned, it is possible to be afraid of anything and, for many, everything. Karl Albrecht, former physicist and now management consultant and author of twenty books, points out five basic fears from which all others originate:[7]

1. Extinction: the fear of being destroyed or no longer existing (i.e., fear of death).

2. Mutilation: the fear of bodily attack or invasion that causes loss of function, mobility, or integrity. This can include the fear of dogs, spiders, and snakes as well as

Figure 3.1
Fear Inventory Prompt List

God	Death	Insanity	Insecurity
Rejection	Intimacy	Diseases	Alcohol
Drugs	Relapse	Sin	Self-expression
Authority	Being found out	Sex	Heights
Unemployment	Employment	Doctors/hospitals	Police/jail
Feelings	Change	Failure	Success
Being alone	Losing a loved one	Physical pain	Drowning
Races	Disapproval	Rejection	Confrontation
Violence	Government	Gossip	Guns

a viral or bacterial infection. It can also include being afraid that something or someone will harm us.

3. Loss of autonomy: the fear of being controlled by a force or person other than us. In the physical form, it is most commonly called claustrophobia and manifests itself as the fear of being held down, enclosed, immobilized, restricted, overwhelmed, captured, imprisoned, or smothered. In the emotional form, it is the fear of certain types of relationships (i.e., fear of intimacy).

4. Separation: the fear of being separated from the herd. It can manifest itself as the fear of abandonment, rejection, and loneliness. It also includes the feeling of not being respected, loved, or valued by others.

5. Ego-death: the fear of any emotional mechanism that can destroy *Self*-integrity, such as humiliation, *Self*-pity, and shame. It can give rise to fears similar to separation but has more to do with damaging our sense of worth.

Consolidating these fears is not simply an academic exercise. It allows us to link seemingly irrational fears to original events when a legitimate fear was born. For example, my fear of loss of control on airplanes can be traced back to a very rational fear of being held down during abuse. They both fit under the category loss of autonomy.

Control Freaks

I believe the greatest fear people struggle with is their lack of control over the future. Incorporated into this fear are all of the five basic fears explained above. No matter how desperate and painful a current situation, many seem to find the status quo less fearful than an uncertain future. As the popular saying goes, "Better the devil you know than the devil you don't."

As I discussed in chapter 1, we are born with a powerful primitive instinct to control our environments. Our early ancestors depended on it to survive. As modern humans, we continue to hold tight to this instinct and particularly the fear of not being in control. However, individuals who resist change and insist on certainty in their future will be unhappy, anxious, and angry most of the time because the future is unpredictable. Change is scary and requires us to have the courage to walk into an undetermined yet potentially beautiful new adventure.

I like what Elliot Cohen, one of the principal founders of philosophical counseling in the United States, says: "It is this contradiction between the demand for certainty and the reality of uncertainty that will continuously play out again and again without resolution, unless you give up the demand for certainty. It is you who must concede; for reality won't give up its uncertainty for you."[8] Unless we give up our will to control the future, the future cannot be different from the present. For some, giving up control happens quickly. For others, particularly those who harbor intense fear(s), it can take a lifetime. Those who continue to feed their fears will have no capacity to surrender control.

I recently spoke to a friend about her decision to leave a physically and emotionally abusive marriage. Janet articulated her thoughts and feelings on what it took to overcome terrifying fears of both her past and her present to move into an uncertain future. I asked her if she would describe this time in her life for the purpose of this book. She courageously agreed, hoping her experience might help others make difficult decisions in their lives.

When I was twelve, my mother left my father and me for another man. She only left a note behind. As an only child whose dad worked long hours as a pharmacist, I spent much of my time alone. I felt unlovable, useless, and not even worthy of a "normal" family like my other friends. If I had been, my mom would have stayed.

Growing up, I wanted to be loved and to have a family, but not just any family. I wanted six kids. I wanted to be a housewife and play the part in my happy family because mine had been torn apart. I figured if I could create this magical family to replace the one that had been destroyed, I would be happy. Everything would be okay again. But that was a lie, a lie I lived for fifteen years.

I ended up in an abusive marriage, one where I was told every day that I was stupid, fat, too religious, a terrible mother, and couldn't do anything right. Still, I scurried around, always trying to make everything "perfect" for my abusive husband in hopes he would love me enough to stick around. Still, I never believed I would be good enough. Throughout our marriage, my husband used drugs, cheated on me, and even physically roughed me up. I ignored these toxic behaviors, choosing instead to pick up the familiar, rumpled bag of denial and wear it over my head. I rationalized the lies my husband told me because I feared being alone and not having anyone take care of me, as had happened to me as a child.

For fifteen years, I kept that bag over my head and created a fictional world for others to see. I focused on family appearance, raising successful children, and painting an overall picture of a happy life. In my heart and behind closed doors, however, I was dying from the illusion and fear of losing everything.

But one day, something happened. A metaphysical nuclear bomb went off. Reality struck down my fictional world, and I realized the rubble I was sitting in. I could deny it no more. My husband had done enough, and I'd had enough. I was faced with a life-altering decision—to leave the marriage or to stay. I had to choose whether to jump off a cliff and lose the identity I had created for so long or continue to bury myself in a destructive life.

Suddenly, I was faced with uncertainty. I no longer knew who I was or what I would do next. The edge of the cliff was a scary place because I didn't know where I would land or how bad the fall would hurt. But to turn away from the cliff meant walking back into the familiar cage and dying. Jump or die?

In the face of uncertainty, I jumped, and I chose life!

I am so grateful for Janet's display of courage to face the unknown. Before I show you how this woman has transformed her life, I would like to point out how devastating childhood experiences often give rise to difficult situations later in life.

Abandoned by her mother, Janet believed she was worthless and unlovable. In addition, because as a child her family had been torn apart, she was driven to re-create an ideal family at any cost.

Consequently, Janet was likely to choose almost anyone who might make her feel loved and give her a family. With low *Self*-esteem, Janet chose a man who was incapable of meeting her emotional needs. Unfortunately, he abused her and her children. In chapter 9, I will explore why we choose certain relationships, particularly unhealthy ones, but it is worth noting here that Janet did nothing to deserve her abuse. Adults thrust neglect upon her as a little girl.

The most vital aspect of Janet's story is that despite all her past and present fears, she found the courage to face them, escape her situation, and change her life. I am amazed to see what her life looks like today, and I am sure you will be too.

This single mother of four recently completed a master's degree in gerontology and is the cofounder of a newly created start-up company that helps people with Alzheimer's disease. Janet has grown from a timid, unsure, and wounded individual ruled by fear of abandonment into a strong, confident woman who loves fully and trusts her *Self* and others. Importantly, her children have greatly benefited from her healthy strength and powerful example of how to move from living under painful dominance and fear into the full light of freedom and beauty. Because of her extraordinary bravery, they are unlikely to replicate similar fear-based behaviors, and they have a great chance of living joyful lives.

We must recognize and realize that our attempts to control life based on System 1 emotions, fears, and reactions end in disaster. For many of us, the worse things get, the more we believe we need to tighten the reins on our chaotic lives, only to experience firsthand the consequences of more confusion and destruction.

I find it fascinating that the phrases "do not be afraid" and "fear not" appear over eighty times in the Bible. Do you think God is trying to tell us something? Clearly, the writers of this sacred text anticipated our natural tendency toward fear, our bent to hold on to the familiar. I realize undoing this grip is hard for many of us, especially when we are inundated with messages in the media, in advertising, and even in everyday conversations that heighten our level of fear to an unhealthy and destructive degree.

Not So Clear and Present Dangers

Global terrorism. Child abductions. School shootings. Carjackings. ISIS. Domestic violence. Murder. Rape. All these words are enough to elicit spine-tingling chills and panic.

I recently dined in a restaurant in my hometown and overheard a conversation at the table next to mine. An elderly gentleman said to his dining companion, "Can you believe all the stuff you hear on the news? I remember how safe it was here forty years ago. We never locked a car or house door. Today I would never take a walk around my block without locking the doors of my house or carrying a gun with me. How did our society go to hell so quickly?"

Would you have agreed with this man?

I find this type of conversation alarming because actual facts reveal nothing could be farther from the truth. Statistics from every category of local and national crime, as well as world violence, indicate we have never been safer nor the planet more peaceful. Recent books (including *Winning the War on War*, *The Tragedy of Great Power Politics*, and *The Better Angels of Our Nature*) document these improvements. In *The Better Angels of Our Nature*, Harvard psychologist Steven Pinker offers powerful data proving a dramatic reduction in war deaths, family violence, racism, rape, and murder. He says, "The decline of violence may be the most significant and least appreciated development in the history of our species."[9]

According to a slew of research Pinker conducted, the number of people dying in global wars has dropped two-hundredfold from the last century until today. Violent crime is markedly down since the 1970s, the time span that my fellow restaurant patron referred to. Since 1976, the rate of domestic murder, husbands killing wives, has decreased almost 50 percent. Rape has dropped over 80 percent since 1973.[10]

In light of these statistics, I was tempted to address the gentleman at the next table and say, "You know, sir, if you didn't lock your doors in the 1970s, I sure wouldn't start locking them now, because in the history of humanity, you have never been safer." Had I chimed in, however, I have a feeling he wouldn't have believed me despite the fact that statistics, derived from several independent sources, could not be clearer. Because System 1 is often highly inaccurate and has little capacity to assess risk, it narrows attention and closes minds to actual facts. No matter the degree of evidence, individuals driven by System 1 fears still believe their assessment of the current situation.

With regard to global terrorism, one of the most highlighted news issues of the day, Pinker points out that "terrorism doesn't account for many deaths. September 11 was just off the scale. There was never a US terrorist attack before or after that had as many deaths. What it does is generate fear."[11] I first want to acknowledge the unimaginable pain that terrorists have inflicted on victims and society because of their unconscionable acts of violence. These are evil deeds perpetrated by evil people. But while many live in constant fear of another act of terrorism being carried out on domestic soil, is this truly a legitimate concern?

A recent study indicates that the chance of the average person in the United States being killed by international terrorists is comparable to the chance of dying by getting struck by an asteroid or drowning in a toilet.[12] So while terrorism exists in the US, whether in the form of ISIS, Boko Haram, or Al-Qaeda, the research reveals that our fear far exceeds the risk from terrorism. We need not constantly worry about our office building, our kids' elementary school, or our neighborhood being blown up.

But fear is nonetheless prevalent. We simply do not have strong enough organizations, information sources, or positive messaging within our culture to effectively slow or disrupt the people, media, and marketers who sell fear.

In a study published in the *Archives of General Psychiatry*, scientists tracked a sample of Americans for a few years post 9/11. They found that 6 percent of those individuals most psychologically impacted by the attacks suffered long-term anxiety and fear and were three times more likely than the remaining 94 percent to have heart problems.[13] If the cited study population is representative of the entire country, this would translate to more than fifteen million people with new heart problems because of their fear of terrorism. If only a small fraction of these people die of a stroke or heart attack, the number killed by fear will still be much higher than the number of 9/11 victims. Fear is devastating and deadly.

Roosevelt nailed it: the only thing we have to fear is fear itself.

System 1 habitually overestimates the degree of actual danger of daily situations. Without cognitive System 2 intervention, our unconscious System 1 will see any horrific event on TV or hear about it from others and assume the event could or will happen to us. It does not matter that the event occurred on the other side of the world in a completely different context. Our System 1 unconsciously and automatically links what we see as a threat to us in the here and now. Since we constantly see and hear about violence and devastation all over the world, few people believe the actual statistics that show the occurrence of crime and world violence is dramatically decreasing.

I notice a trend among some leaders in certain faith communities. Many push fear from behind a podium so parishioners recognize that we are in the last days before the coming apocalypse and will therefore be motivated to embrace the spiritual life. These religious leaders tend to instill the fear of God into whoever is listening by citing stories and showing videos of violent acts perpetrated around the globe. Not only is fear an ineffective means to change people, but it is also counterproductive. It generates more anxiety, more stress, and more stress-related illnesses in others. I would say to these leaders, "Stop pushing fear and instead proclaim peace and love from Christ."

I believe the Scriptures' warning that there will one day be a second coming of Jesus. But he reminds us, "About that day or hour no one knows, not even the angels in heaven, nor the Son, but only the Father" (Matt. 24:36). While Jesus provided signs foretelling his return, including horrific wars, turmoil, natural disasters, and moral decline—and we see evidence of these things in modern-day society—from a purely mathematical perspective, the frequency of activities described in these signs has never been lower. Of course this could change, but for now violent death rates, for instance, are over a thousandfold lower than when the second coming was prophesied. I hope this encourages you to align your *Self* with the recurring theme of the Bible to "fear not."

The Damage of Unsubstantiated Fear

Opening our *Selves* to fear-inducing publications, media, and even people (by habitually watching twenty-four-hour news networks, tuning into satellite radio talk shows, or repeating the same conversations with others about how terrible, unsafe, and violent our world is) causes more catastrophic damage than we can imagine.

From a science and genetics (a primary focus in my research) perspective, environmental stimulants that evoke fear structurally alter our brain DNA. A special subcategory of genetics known as epigenetics is one of the fastest-growing disciplines in science. It studies how our environments (everything from exposure to psychological challenges to our diets) change the very structure of our DNA. Though I discuss this in great detail in the next chapter, for now just know that fear is a major factor that alters the DNA in our brains and that leads to brain rewiring.

Specifically, trauma and fear create stress, which alters our DNA, turns up certain genes in our brains, and ultimately creates fear-based nerve connections. All of this fear-based brain wiring then keeps us constantly afraid and anxious. Tragically, fear also leads to stress-associated changes in other parts of our bodies that eventually cause pathologies such as high blood pressure and inflammation. That is why fear produced by 9/11 caused so much heart disease.

Consequently, if we fill our minds with copious amounts of fear-producing stimuli (such as advertising, twenty-four-hour news cycles, and fear-based politics), stress created by this fear interacts with genes in our brain cells to make fear-based pathways stronger. We then pay a heavy price, the cost of developing mental and physical ailments such as paranoia, anxiety, depression, heart disease, and stroke.

Each year I spend several weeks in isolated regions of Africa where I have no access to any kind of media. I am always amazed when I get back to the States that nothing has changed.

I return home to the same global conflicts, the same religious disputes, the same pain and suffering, the same weather "storms of the century." Republicans and Democrats; liberals and conservatives; powers in the Middle East, the United States, and Russia; atheists and believers still battle. Wolf Blitzer still ominously opens every CNN telecast with "we now have important breaking news," as if you and your family are at great risk unless you hear the upcoming story. This brings to mind King Solomon's words in the ancient text of Ecclesiastes that "generations come and generations go, but the earth never changes" (1:4 NLT).

Here is a helpful tool if you want to significantly reduce your fear and create more joy in your life starting today: decrease your consumption of fear-based stimuli. Turn off the TV and especially twenty-four-hour news feeds. Listen to uplifting music on your car rides. Refuse to accept as fact much of the unsubstantiated information you are continually fed from your environment. Politely end conversations that focus on doom and gloom.

I am not saying you should make like Pollyanna and pretend that evil or bad people and things do not exist. I am offering that you stop bingeing on fear-based information so you can decrease fear-based circuits in your brain that destroy your happiness and health. This is one simple and relatively easy way to begin to rewire your brain and quickly experience more joy in your life.

The Choice to Change

This chapter contains some heavy content, and I will end it on an encouraging note. However powerful your fear-based brain circuits are, you can choose not to be afraid or indulge in unfounded fear. I have spent much of my life afraid of being happy. There was something in me that unconsciously and repeatedly sent the message to my brain that I was not worthy of being happy. This fear almost destroyed my ability to laugh, play, and have fun.

My father was the freest man I ever knew, and good or bad, if he thought something, he said or did it. I can remember that everything was always the best. He ate the "best" pie, watched the "best" sunset, and enjoyed the "best" day at the beach. A burgeoning scientist at the time, I felt it my job one day to challenge him. I often told him, in what I am embarrassed to admit was a bit of a snarky tone, "Well, Dad, statistically it's impossible for everything to be the best." My father simply smiled in response. I am sure he felt sorry for me in that moment and probably thought something like, "Oh, dear son. You just don't get it, do you?"

No, Dad, I didn't.

Because my father lived only in the now, the pie, the sunset, and the day at the beach really were the best he ever had. There was no past to compare it to. He did not live in yesterday, bound by fears or haunting experiences. He lived for today. In time and in his passing, I came to realize that Dad lived life the right way, free and fearless. This is exactly how we all are meant, created, to live.

Seventeen years ago, I gave the eulogy at my father's funeral. In my talk, I made a promise to spend the rest of my life with the goal of living as freely and as fearlessly as my father. Today those who are close to me would say I am definitely on that journey. I often hear people quietly comment while shaking their heads, "That Ski Chilton is one crazy man." I just smile and think, "Dad, you would be proud of me. I'm getting there!" I am not afraid of being happy anymore. Enjoying this freedom has been one of the most life-changing transformations in my life.

It takes courage to explore our fears and the System 1 dysfunctions that have made our lives unmanageable. I love the line in Shakespeare's *Julius Caesar* where the Roman leader says to his wife as the noise of battle approaches and dying men and ghosts shriek in the streets, "Cowards die many times before their deaths: the valiant never taste of death but once."[14]

Our constant worry about yesterday and our fear of tomorrow diminish and destroy our capacity to be present in the moment, to be joyful, to live free. But once we find the courage and the desire within us to change, we can discover *Self*-directed paths that override System 1 dysfunctions. We can overcome our most pressing fears. We can be intentional in our thoughts and actions. We cannot die a thousand deaths thinking about them.

Reflection: The Pathway to Rewire Your Mind

1. Do you believe fear affects your everyday feelings and decisions? If so, how? Who do you become when you are overwhelmed with fear?

2. What is the most important area of your life in which fear is holding you back? Use the "Fear Inventory Prompt List" shown earlier in this chapter to help you assess what makes you nervous, anxious, and afraid.

3. How much do you expose your *Self* to fear-based stimuli (such as advertising, news cycles, certain religious

practices, etc.)? What is one thing you can do starting today to lower your exposure?

4. Given the huge misconceptions Americans can have about the risk of a given situation, what is the one area of your life in which you have most overestimated the risk of something bad happening?

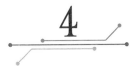

Your Brain on Change

Growth is the only evidence of life.

John Henry Newman,
Apologia pro vita sua, 1864

In 1997, Cheryl Schiltz woke up one morning and fell out of bed. Feeling dizzy, she thought her bedroom looked lopsided, and she struggled unsuccessfully to regain her balance. This strange sensation never went away.

Tests showed Cheryl's vestibular system, the canals in the inner ear that coordinate balance and tell us up from down, was destroyed. Doctors offered no hope. While they pinpointed the source of the problem, a severe side effect from an antibiotic she had taken following a recent surgery, there was nothing they could do. Cheryl was destined to stagger around like a drunk, falling over and clinging to walls for stability.

A few years later, she volunteered for an experimental study conducted by Paul Bach-y-Rita, a neuroscientist in the University of Wisconsin Medical School's orthopedics and rehabilitation department. Bach-y-Rita had long argued that the sensory part of the brain could readapt to devastating losses. He fitted Cheryl with a hard hat that contained a device called an accelerometer, which was wired to a strip of tape containing 144 microelectrodes that he placed on her tongue. The accelerometer communicated her spatial coordinates to a computer, which in turn fed the information to the strip that buzzed on her tongue.

The first time she wore the hat Cheryl cried out of sheer joy; the debilitating feeling of falling disappeared. She could balance without needing the two canes she relied on to walk as straight as possible, which was not anywhere near how we define straight. Cheryl wore the hat for a few minutes each day while Bach-y-Rita buzzed her tongue, stimulating the sensory regions of her brain. As time passed, whenever she removed the hat, her sense of balance would remain intact for a few minutes before the wobbling set in. This residual stability increased the longer she wore the hat over the course of a year. Eventually, Cheryl regained total balance without needing the device.

What happened? As a result of the stimulations Cheryl's tongue received, her brain rewired itself by creating new nerve connections, thus completely recovering her vestibular system. This is powerful stuff! Especially when you consider that medical professionals had basically given up on her, relying on long-standing scientific theories that the brain cannot change.

What We First Believed

Scientists initially believed that the brain was a physiologically static organ; once a human being reached adulthood, brain structure was fixed. The number of brain cells (neurons) you had was largely determined by your genetics, and these neurons were arranged in a certain unchangeable architecture by early childhood experiences. The patterns of connections between the neurons produced an inflexible set of brain functions, behavioral tendencies, feelings, and thoughts that could not change.

According to this theory, the formation of new neurons, what is called neurogenesis, stopped shortly after birth. To make things worse, it was also generally accepted that not only was it impossible to form new neurons, but a human being also lost tens of thousands of neurons each day. By the age of eighteen, you were who you were. The only way your brain could change was if it was damaged by a stroke or other injury. In that case, whatever part was impaired or destroyed could not be regenerated and was lost forever.

Based on this model, an individual had limited or no capacity to make free choices with regard to their behavior or emotions. It is no wonder we have the cliché "You can't teach an old dog new tricks." As a scientist, I have always wondered who tests the ideas behind such clichés. Is it even possible to measure them? This may sound like trite scrutiny, but I believe certain unsubstantiated clichés can be harmful to society, such as the case of the old dog. This statement conveys a doctrinal message to adults that you are emotionally and behaviorally stuck where you are; you do not have the capacity to make meaningful and positive changes in your life.

Recent discoveries demonstrating the brain's incredible ability to reorganize, rewire, and in many cases repair its architecture, as seen in Cheryl's case, refute the old cliché. In order to better understand and appreciate the beauty of this process known as neuroplasticity, we will delve a little deeper into the science.

The Power of Plasticity

Throughout medical history, there were critics of the static brain theory who believed not only that an old dog can learn new tricks but also that an old dog can teach himself new tricks. Dating back to 350 BC, the brilliant philosopher and scientist Aristotle postulated that creatures change as a result of their internal and external environments throughout their lives and that this change is not accidental. He believed that individual organic forms gradually emerge from the unformed.[1] In 1890, the great philosopher and psychologist William James wrote that "organic matter, especially nervous tissue, seems endowed with a very extraordinary degree of plasticity."[2] Unfortunately, these brilliant men and other scientists who shared the controversial view that the brain had, in fact, the capacity to change were largely ignored until the 1960s.

Around that time researchers began to provide compelling evidence in support of neuroplasticity, also known as brain plasticity, outside of early development. For instance, in 1969, J. S. Griffith and H. R. Mahler proposed that adaptability in brain DNA played a key role in the capacity to retain long-term memory.[3] Their work suggested that there are dynamic changes in the structure of brain DNA throughout life that create specific patterns of brain circuitry necessary to store memories. In other words, a brain's DNA and structure continually develop based on events that occur in a person's life. These observations opened a floodgate of new studies and research that indicated our brains are constantly changing.

This occurs not only after injury but also in response to interactions with our external and internal environments and our experiences, thoughts, and choices. By the 1980s, studies from every discipline of biology and medicine began to show that as organisms, including human beings, interacted with certain environments, the very chemical structure of their DNA actually changed as a result of those interactions. This process is known as epigenetics. I find it an astonishing testament to the brilliance of Aristotle, who proposed this process twenty-four hundred years earlier.

These new understandings emphasize the incredible adaptability of humans. The flexibility of the brain makes us remarkable and truly complex. Norman Doidge is a psychiatrist who has spent many years examining research on neuroplasticity from the best, cutting-edge neurology researchers in the world. He documented this work in his internationally bestselling book *The Brain That Changes Itself*. Doidge wrote:

> I met a scientist who enabled people who had been blind since birth to begin to see, another who enabled the deaf to hear; I spoke with people who had had strokes decades before and had been declared incurable, who were helped to recover with neuroplastic treatments; I met people whose learning disorders were cured and whose IQs were raised; I saw evidence that it is possible for eighty-year-olds to sharpen their memories to function the way they did when they were fifty-five. I saw people rewire their brains with their thoughts, to cure previously incurable obsessions and traumas.[4]

Amazing!

In a bit, I will get to the nuts and bolts of brain architecture and how changes to DNA can alter our behavioral and emotional fates, but right now take in the good news: we can change at any age. Our brains are not fixed or hardwired. If we choose, we can be continuous and beautiful works in progress.

The Fundamentals of Brain Wiring

As you know, early childhood life experiences play a critical role in building the architecture of our brains. During this period of time, billions of neurons build connections called synapses and send signals that allow these brain cells to communicate with one another. As certain neurons interact more often with neighboring neurons, information highways called brain circuits or neural networks are formed. Our life experiences; family, social, and cultural environments; thoughts; and feelings determine which circuits get the most use and which do not.

Connections that are used most get stronger, and much larger circuits are built around them. In contrast, connections that are not used fade away through a process called pruning. Basically, use it or lose it. Or as neuroscientists like to say, "Neurons that fire together, wire together."

I was in Los Angeles a few weeks ago driving on the busiest highway in the United States, the fourteen-lane Interstate 405. Navigating this roadway can be quite a challenge for a country boy like me. Known by city residents as "the 405," this interstate serves about 379,000 vehicles a day.[5] That's a lot of people, goods, and freight moving from one place to another for any one driver to handle.

Imagine your strongest brain circuits as mega-superhighways, the 405 times ten, carrying millions of nerve signals from one

Figure 4.1
System 1 in Overdrive

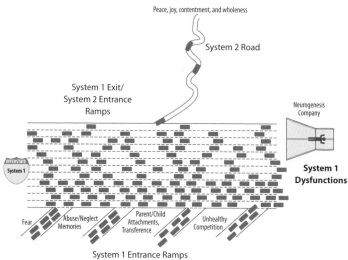

brain location to another each day. Now imagine a highway construction company called Neurogenesis. This company constructs larger superhighways and provides more lanes, new entrance ramps, and better bridges based on the use of a particular highway. The more it is used, the more it gets. Alternatively, if a highway is used less, it receives no additional construction funding and in fact becomes abandoned and eventually deteriorates. What I have just described is a simplified version of how new nerve circuits (highways) are formed and deconstructed.

In more personal terms, if you spend years studying a second language and suddenly stop learning and practicing it, those once strong circuits will weaken and eventually fade away. However, if you continue to develop your foreign tongue, those neural networks will grow even stronger. This applies to many life areas, including emotional dysfunctions.

Figure 4.2
A Balanced System 1/2 Response

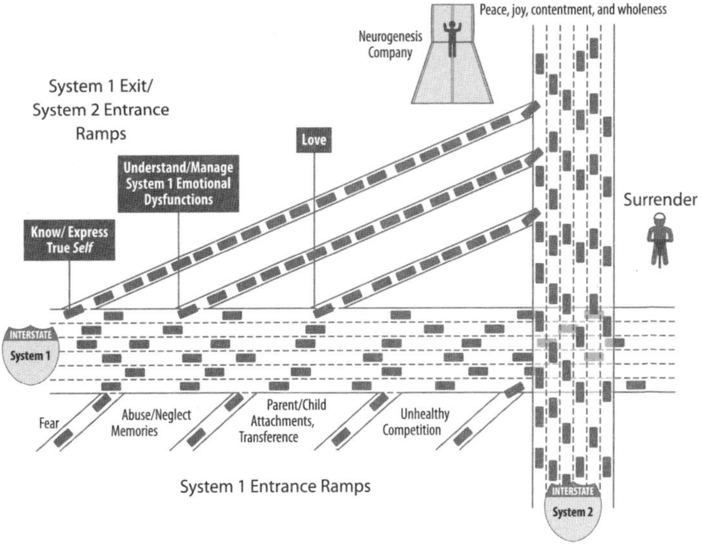

If your System 1 response of anger is out of control, the more you "practice" or engage in road rage, the stronger the neural circuits will be for that particular dysfunction. On the other hand, the more you disengage or override that System 1 response, the more you destroy that particular circuit.

Figure 4.1 shows what your brain is like with System 1 in overdrive. Your System 1 dysfunctions are like a twelve-lane superhighway as you react automatically to most situations. There are wide and well-traveled on-ramps from fear, negative memories, transference, and unhealthy competition. (We will discuss transference in chapter 9.) The off-ramp to System 2 is a sparsely traveled dirt road. Sadly, this is the picture for far too many people.

By contrast, Figure 4.2 shows what a balanced brain looks like, with both System 1 and System 2 functioning properly.

We will unpack this image more in future chapters, but for now just notice that System 1 has fewer lanes, the System 1 off-ramps to System 2 are wide and well traveled, and System 2 itself has as many lanes as System 1.

The Role of Genetics and Environment in Wiring the Brain

I want to be clear that our brains are among the most complex entities in the universe. While scientists understand the basics, the functionality of certain areas of this magnificent organ remains a mystery. As discussed above, we are only beginning to learn how the brain coordinates more than 80 billion neurons to form the architecture of 125 trillion nerve connections in the neocortex alone that produce our behaviors, our thoughts, and our sense of *Self*. To wrap our minds around such complexity, we scientists must come up with simple models so that we can understand this complexity and explain it to others. I use these throughout the book because I believe it is important to envision complex processes using simple analogies.

I will start with a very simple model that I have often used to describe the interaction between genetics and brain plasticity over a lifetime. I compare the development of a brain, including brain plasticity over a lifetime, to the building of a house.

A child inherits his or her genes from two parents. These genes are packaged together to create what is called a structural genome, the essential blueprints that form a human being. The structural genome builds every cell in the body and thus is the critical underpinning for practically every physical, cognitive, and behavioral characteristic a person will ever have. I call the structural genome the "foundational genetics" because this set of blueprints is put in place at the beginning of life, and, barring a rare mutation, the basic information it provides does not change. Information in the blueprints orchestrates assembly of the foundational elements of the brain, the house in my model.

When building a house, an initial set of blueprints is required to construct the basic structure. If there is a good design and the basic structure for the house (including the foundation, framing, roofing, plumbing, and electrical work) is properly carried out, the house has the potential to become a well-built and functional home. However, if the foundation is not on firm footing, the framing is not square, or water leaks from shoddy plumbing, there is a good chance the completed home will have fundamental problems immediately or in the future.

Likewise, if you get a well-designed set of blueprints from the structural genome for your brain, you will have the capacity to develop a life in a wide variety of positive directions; if not, you have a greater risk of developing a mental illness and/or mental deficits.

In house construction, foundational work as set in the initial blueprints is followed by the finishing work, which includes the installation of windows and doors, flooring, painting, landscaping, and interior design. Options are abundant in this stage, and they are determined by factors such as climate, purpose, and personal taste. For example, although they may share similar foundational characteristics, a house in the sweltering Arizona desert will have qualities that differ from those of a house in snowy and cold Alaska. If mistakes or damage from bad weather occur at any of these latter steps, though they may not destroy the structure, they can certainly reduce the functionality and beauty of the home, and it will not become what it was intended to become.

The adaptation of the initial blueprints for finishing work is analogous to epigenetics. All of the changes made to the structural genome are collectively called the epigenome, what I call our "changeable genetics." As a human experiences life, thinks, and makes choices, alterations are made in the brain, including modifications to circuitry that eventually lead to later responses, reactions, and emotions. Just as homeowners have the power to arrange a house to their liking (a neglectful mess, a hoarder's paradise, clutter-free, or spotless and immaculate), your past experiences and responses to them can quite literally change the blueprints, resulting in your present feelings, habits, thoughts, and behaviors.

In summary: Most of us were born with a firm genetic foundation leading to a perfectly good brain. Your parents may not have been the best parents or made the best decisions, but the genes they gave you at conception were strong enough to build a good life.

Then, stuff happened. You endured a traumatic situation out of your control that began to change the blueprints to alter your genetics and, consequently, the internal wiring of your brain. A family member may have abused you verbally, emotionally, or sexually. Maybe your parents went through a nasty divorce. Perhaps you lost a loved one, witnessed a horrific event, or bounced around from foster home to foster home.

These environmental stimuli and their subsequent impacts on your DNA may have forged wiring to regions of your brain that constantly produce fear and anxiety. As a result, you developed heavily trafficked superhighways that carry millions of nerve signals to regions of your brain that create emotional dysfunctions. These dysfunctions may compromise your ability to have intimate relationships; intensify an addictive tendency to abuse alcohol, food, or sex; or cause you to act out emotionally in ways that lead to disastrous outcomes. Sadly, your brain developed a System 1 dysfunctional future based on past negative experiences, feelings, and environments—in other words, a future based on past memories. And this may be where you are today.

What We Think Matters

I think the most revolutionary aspect of brain plasticity is the fact that not only external experiences but also our very thoughts themselves can change our brain wiring. I am fascinated by the work of Jeffrey Schwartz, a practicing neuro-psychiatrist and author of several books, including *Brainlock: Free Yourself from Obsessive-Compulsive Behavior*. Schwartz has had great success treating one of the most intractable mental disorders, obsessive-compulsive disorder (OCD), by helping his patients change the way they think about their feelings and behaviors. Their very thoughts, not drugs, override their default responses, rewire their brains, and eventually permanently change their behavior. OCD is a difficult setting in which to alter behavior, so Schwartz's work offers great hope that we all have the capacity to change dysfunctional behaviors by thinking differently.

I like what Norman Doidge says in his book *The Brain That Changes Itself*: "Imagining an act engages the same motor and sensory programs that are involved in doing it. We have long viewed our imaginative life with a kind of sacred awe: as noble, pure, immaterial, and ethereal, cut off from our material brain. Now we cannot be so sure about where to draw the line between them."[6]

Our thought life is powerful. Actions, good and bad, result from what we think about. I love what the Episcopal bishop John Beckwaith said in the nineteenth century:

> Plant a thought and reap a word;
> plant a word and reap an action;
> plant an action and reap a habit;
> plant a habit and reap a character;
> plant a character and reap a destiny.[7]

If you want to become a more generous person, you must push your *Self* to regularly do good things for others. If you start down that path, over time you will become a generous person. If you tell your *Self*, "I'm not a generous person. It's just not in my nature," then you will continue to give to others sparingly. As Beckwaith says above, we become the type of people our thoughts tell us to be.

When you have a thought that you repeatedly act upon, your thoughts and resultant actions become a habit. Through this process you direct your brain to change its wiring. Repetition of the same thoughts, actions, and habits strengthens the wiring to make the habit more powerful. While the System 1 emotional dysfunctions we have discussed are hardwired in your brain, you can weaken them by not using them and build new wiring to a better place by thinking differently.

Because your thoughts matter, it is important to learn to be careful with them. Do not compromise your *Self*. With time and practice, be conscious of any negative or *Self*-destructive thoughts because they highly influence who you are and who you will become. In light of our new understanding of genetics and its relationship to brain plasticity, System 1 emotional dysfunctions and negative *Self*-talk take on a whole new meaning. In this context, this means you can change your DNA and thus your future. Thinking the same negative or unhealthy thoughts will reap an unhealthy and negative destiny.

Fortunately, recent science in positive psychology and cognitive behavioral therapies suggests that the converse is also true. You can plant positive thoughts of change and reap not only a positive brain DNA change but also positive altered brain wiring, actions, character, and ultimately a positive future.

I have heard several variations of the following story: "A Native American elder once described his own inner struggles in this manner: Inside of me there are two dogs. One of the dogs is mean and evil. The other dog is good. The mean dog fights the good dog all the time. When asked which dog wins, he reflected for a moment and replied, The one I feed the most."[8]

Because of brain plasticity, the thoughts we feed the most get stronger. Want to change your life and your mind? Change your thoughts. (I offer more direction on how to do so in part 3 of this book). I want to encourage you that even right now you are in the center of change. By simply reading this book, four chapters in, you are beginning to understand that you may have been feeding the wrong dog.

Here is the most important and exciting news of this book: you own your mind and can choose how to focus your thoughts. Because of the wonders of brain plasticity, your

Self-directed thoughts, choices, and actions can change your brain and your mind. But this takes desire, practice, many new starts, and courage to work hard.

Pay close attention to the latter part of what I just wrote.

The Capacity to Change

Though I have said and studies have shown that anyone, regardless of age, can change, the reality is that not everyone has the capacity to do so. Before you accuse me of making a contradictory statement, hear me out.

Chapter 5 of AA's *The Big Book* says that "those who do not recover are people who cannot or will not completely give themselves to this simple program, usually men and women who are constitutionally incapable of being honest with themselves."[9]

From a scientific and philosophical perspective, I am fascinated by this observation, particularly by the words "constitutionally incapable." At the time of this writing, I have submitted a paper to *Neuroethics* describing a new genetic and philosophical model of moral development. I describe how we are born with free will, or, as it is called in philosophical circles, the principle of alternative possibilities. Basically, this is just a fancy way of saying we were created constitutionally capable of choosing our actions in a given situation. Sadly, many appear to lose this. Let me explain. At the risk of overgeneralizing, I believe most humans fall into one of three categories in this regard.

The first group is completely driven by their survival of the fittest instincts. Their responses in most situations are firmly wired and completely predictable. They operate by competition, selfishness, *Self*-admiration, and control in any environment at any cost. They typically live by the motto "The one who dies with the most toys wins" and will fight anything or anyone who gets in their way.

Picture, if you will, the narcissist. This person lacks the capacity to express empathy for others and pays little attention to moral codes or values. This approach is applied to all aspects of life, including relationships, careers, and social settings. It is extraordinarily difficult for this person to reflect on their life or change course. From a neuroscience perspective, I believe anyone in this category has permanently wired their brain circuitry in a manner that is almost certainly unchangeable.

The second group consists of basically decent folks who are also resistant to *Self*-examination, reflection, and honesty. This is C. S. Lewis's "gradual slope" people. They, like most of us, have been hurt and typically react to their environments in an instinctive or fear-based manner. These responses consistently result in negative feelings and behaviors.

The "gradual slope" people unconsciously repeat the same mistakes, the same unhealthy cycles, and the same toxic relationship patterns. However, they are stuck because they do not ever consider their own contributions to their situations. They do not believe they have a problem, much less admit they are the problem.

For these people, everyone else is to blame. For instance, a man may repeatedly choose to date unhealthy women who toy with his emotions and even cheat on him. While he may be right and can make a great case that the mates he selects are not good people, he somehow misses the fact that he is ultimately responsible for picking the same type of toxic person over and over.

The people in this group adapt and live with their desperation. It usually takes a dramatic and painful experience to wake them up from their manageable existence. Change is difficult. It is easier and much safer not to ask or answer the difficult questions and stay stuck.

Individuals in the third group have also suffered from this broken world. They have made mistakes, hurt others, and experienced great pain and devastation as a result of their unconscious responses to trauma, abuse, rejection, neglect, and betrayal at some point in their lives.

However, unlike the former groups, they are keenly and painfully aware that many of their strategies and approaches to life have not worked, and they are determined to find new and better ways to find and express their true *Selves* and transition away from their destructive responses and situations. They have lost in life, but they have not given up. They have a strong desire to learn new ways to live in order to create a better future.

You are a part of this group. You recognize and acknowledge your life needs to change. And now that you understand the power you and your thoughts have to change your brain genetics and brain wiring, you are ready to continue on the path of making better choices and living fearlessly. You are ready to learn how.

I believe God was well aware of how tough this earthly life would be and therefore deemed it essential to provide us with minds that can recover from our deepest hurts and mistakes. In this way, he made it possible for us to get second, third, and more chances at a new life.

That being said, the process of rewiring is not easy. The circuits and superhighways developed by our past must be downgraded and new, more powerful ones built. Without specific strategies to accomplish this, change is not likely. We cannot simply will our brains to function in a more healthy and positive way; we have to work for it. We have to learn. We have to practice.

If you ignore and simply hope destructive mind highways of the past will disappear, they and all the System 1 dysfunctions associated with them will only get stronger. However, if you, your true *Self*, deeply desire change and are willing to practice specific strategies to accomplish this goal, these pathways to disastrous outcomes will weaken and eventually atrophy. You may not be able to immediately stop being controlling, fearful, sad, or angry, but the goal is to use these roadways less and less and more quickly locate the exit ramps to new, positive thoughts and behaviors.

While the insight you gain and the questions you answer at the end of each chapter will help move you toward rewiring your mind, the third part of this book, particularly the exercises, will help guide, direct, and reinforce this process.

After I hit my emotional bottom and began to change my life (detailed more fully in chapter 12), I painted every room in my house a bright Mediterranean color and placed new, vivid art in each one. This interior design transformation was symbolic of the positive changes I chose to make in my mind. I am not naïve. I know that changing my life—getting rid of the cycle of System 1 dysfunctions, addictive patterns, and fear-based choices—requires a lot more than a fresh coat of paint and some eye-catching pictures.

I believe transformations of great magnitude require hope, great courage, deep faith, and, as the AA program advocates, "a searching and fearless" inventory of our behaviors. This is no easy task. Remember, AA encourages a "one day at a time" philosophy. This principle is designed to encourage the recovering addict not to be overwhelmed by the thought of staying sober for a lifetime but to focus only on the present day. This outlook makes the recovery process more manageable. Because change is so hard, for beginners to the program, the motto is often modified to "one minute at a time." When you strive to rewire your brain, it is crucial to adopt this idea. Don't set your *Self* up for failure by expecting to change your brain wiring and weaken or destroy your System 1 dysfunctions overnight. Take this process one step, one day, one hour, one minute at a time. If you are committed, you will see the process of change happen over time. Not tomorrow or next week, but it can happen!

Reflection: The Pathway to Rewire Your Mind

1. How often have you described someone as being unable to change? In other words, when have you said, "He is who he is and will always be that way." In light of the information you read in this chapter, how do you view your previous statements?

2. Does the idea that your very thoughts can change the basic architecture of your brain motivate you to strive for a better future? What encourages or discourages you?

3. Can you identify some of your patterns of negative thinking, feelings, and reactions that are constant and may very well be part of a brain circuit superhighway?

4. What expectations do you have at this very moment as far as rewiring your brain? Describe your level of commitment.

PART 2

REFRAME

Here we help you face reality and determine ways to put into perspective and deal with some of the more pressing and specific issues in life. We will begin these explorations by offering a preliminary look at our human condition to help you understand what it means to be human and the importance of morality. Then you will have the opportunity to learn the different approaches many of us take and need to adapt in areas including:

tragedy and trauma
parenting
relationships
sex and intimacy

While we will help you evaluate your behaviors in the different areas of your life, we encourage you to supplement your learning by seeking outside counseling (via a counselor, a professional spiritual advisor like a pastor, a mentor, or a support group) for your areas of intense struggle.

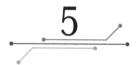

What It Means to Be Human

> This awareness of himself as a separate entity, the
> awareness of his own short life span, of the fact
> that without his will he is born and against his
> will he dies, that he will die before those whom
> he loves, or they before him, the awareness of
> his aloneness and separateness, of his helpless-
> ness before the forces of nature and of society,
> all this makes his separate, disunited existence
> an unbearable prison.
>
> Erich Fromm, *The Art of Loving*

I can still picture my dad walking into the house after a long
day's work out in the tobacco fields. Mopping his sweaty
forehead with a dusty handkerchief, he would plant himself
at the dinner table with a smile, much to the delight of my
two sisters and me. After our bellies were full with Mom's

mouthwatering meal, Daddy would mosey into the living room and load a large stack of 45 rpm records on our RCA Victor record player. As the sun set, he would lie on the cool floor and close his eyes, his toes rhythmically tapping in the air to the sounds of soul music. On any given day, the smooth voices of the Temptations, Otis Redding, Aretha Franklin, Marvin Gaye, and the Supremes would croon from the record player until the sky was pitch-black and crickets chirped.

We kids loved this part of evenings. Even though Detroit, the home of Motown, was seemingly a million miles away in distance and culture, my daddy introduced me to rhythm and blues heaven right there in rural North Carolina. We would dance to the beat of the scratchy music and do our best impressions of James Brown, a tough feat for a little white boy from a tobacco farm. There was something about those tunes that made tough days end almost magically. I remember one day asking Dad why he loved soul music so much. He said to me, "Ski, soul artists sing about their feelings. They show you what's in their hearts. And they tell you the truth about life."

I still love Motown. So does my son Josh, who lives with me. Every morning as we get ready for work, we blast our classic soul and R & B Pandora stations. I always think with a smile, "Daddy, you would be so proud. Your musical legacy lives on in both your son and your grandson."

During the writing of this chapter, I woke up one morning and, as I always do, turned on my iPad and tuned into Pandora's "Old Soul Radio" station. A desperate refrain from a 1974 song covered by Main Ingredient repeated itself incessantly through the speakers: "I just don't want to be lonely." As I brushed my teeth, I struggled with what to write for this particular chapter. My thoughts centered on the complexity of our extraordinary human minds that makes System 2 reasoning possible and makes us unique in all of creation. Over the last several days, I had been deep in the process of gathering content but had struggled with the enormous weight of the question "What does it mean to be human?"

Toothbrush in hand, I stared at my reflection in the mirror as I contemplated all of the different aspects of the human condition. Was it possible to sum up the essence of human existence in one chapter, in light of over four thousand years of literature on this topic?

In the midst of these thoughts, the previously dulled melodies of the first song of the day sounded louder than my introspection. And suddenly, the significance of the song and particularly the refrain came into focus. What it means to be human is to struggle with anguishing isolation, a desperate need to be in relationships, and an often-tumultuous journey to find a solution to our loneliness.

First Principles

This chapter marks the onset of the second part of this book. Before we begin to reframe the most important parts of our lives, I believe it is critical that we understand the baseline of our human condition. What is the essence of a human being that ultimately influences and even dictates how and why we need to reframe the imbalances or chaos in our lives?

I love to think of this in terms of "first principles," which the *Oxford English Dictionary* defines as "the fundamental concepts or assumptions on which a theory, system, or method is based."[1] Elon Musk, founder of SpaceX and cofounder of Zip2, PayPal, and Tesla Motors, says what this really means is "that you boil things down to the most fundamental truths and then reason up from there."[2]

Some of the greatest inventors of our time, such as Elon Musk, now believe that understanding first principles is the foundation of the most important and life-changing creativity, thoughts, and innovations. Trained as a biochemist, I was taught that it is not until we have some capacity to discern how something works at its most basic level that we can initiate change or innovation in a meaningful way.

Once we better understand the human condition, obviously an ambitious task to attempt in one chapter, we will be better able to view our lives and their different facets within the context of that lens. I must point out that this subject is not a System 1 or a System 2 issue. The human condition lies at the center of these two forces as it defines the most fundamental issues of existence. That said, I am going to suspend a lot of the System 1 / System 2 language to focus primarily on what it means to be human.

Our Human Condition

I am going to probe this topic from two perspectives: a biblical one and a scientific one. First, let's analyze what the Bible reveals about our human condition and particularly the relationship between God and humankind from the beginning of time.

A Biblical Perspective

We read in the first book of the Bible that God said:

"Let us make mankind in our image, in our likeness, so that they may rule over the fish in the sea and the birds in the sky,

over the livestock and all the wild animals, and over all the
creatures that move along the ground."
So God created mankind in his own image, in the image
of God he created them; male and female he created them.
(Gen. 1:26–27)

This ancient text, which sits at the foundation of Christianity, Judaism, and Islam, links humans to God as his mirror image.

So what does it mean to be like God? The description
of God provided not only by these verses but by the entire
book of Genesis gives us an important snapshot of who
he is and thus who we are in his image. First, we have been
given an incredible capacity to reason, think, and create
that far surpasses that of any animal. Evidenced through
art, music, literature, medicine, technology, and architecture, we see God's image reflected in human creativity and
intelligence.

Second, the single most important trait that we share with
God is that we are relational. God, as depicted throughout
the Bible, has a deep desire to communicate with and have a
relationship with humankind. And yet he has given us incredible brains with the mental and spiritual capacity to choose
to reciprocate the sentiment. We are not automatons coerced
into loving or engaging with him.

Clearly, a central tenet of God's relational nature is freedom. This is represented by the tree of knowledge of good
and evil in the Garden of Eden (Gen. 2:9, 17). God gave
Adam and Eve full access to the natural food supply of this
utopic land, save for one tree. Although he was clear in his
instruction that they refrain from indulging their appetites
on the fruits of this particular tree, God also gave Adam

and Eve the free will to disobey. It was apparent from the beginning that love and obedience had no meaning to God unless given freely.

But freedom and especially disobedience come at a terrible cost. C. S. Lewis says, "The lost enjoy forever the horrible freedom they have demanded."[3] This was powerfully illustrated after Adam and Eve tasted the fruit from the forbidden tree. After this act of rebellion, "their eyes were opened, and they suddenly felt shame at their nakedness" (Gen. 3:7 NLT). At that moment, Adam and Eve became aware of themselves and their separateness as individuals. They also realized, with great pain, that they were now separated from God.

According to Erich Fromm, "The awareness of human separation, without reunion by love—is the source of shame. It is at the same time the source of guilt and anxiety. The deepest need of man, then, is the need to overcome his separateness, to leave the prison of his aloneness."[4] Adam and Eve had not yet learned to love or relate to each other, as evidenced by the fact that after God questioned what they had done, Adam responded with a very System 1 move. Rather than defending Eve, he blamed her for causing him to eat the fruit.

As with us today, their unwise use of free will created a chasm between themselves and God and even between the two of them, as they were aware for the first time that they were alone. The incredible truth found in Scripture is that the destructive use of freedom separates us from God and each other. Freedom is so powerful because it contains both true love and true evil. Depending on our choices, it is the ultimate source of our union and joy as well as our separateness and pain.

Throughout the Bible, we see God's plan to reestablish union and relationship with humankind through covenants with key individuals like Abraham, Noah, and David. As Christians, we believe our ultimate reunification with God comes through our trust in and our connection and covenant with his Son, Jesus Christ.

As a father of four adult children who were at times, quite frankly, hellions to parent, I am drawn to God's response to Adam and Eve's disobedience. He first admonishes them with a powerful rebuke. Then, knowing they have lost their innocence and have been burdened with the painful loneliness of being separated from him for the rest of their lives, God shows them remarkable compassion and unconditional love. Before he sends them off into the world, he makes them new clothes to cover their naked bodies (Gen. 3:21). This picture brings tears to my eyes. In this passage, I see God as a parent who is not so different from me. When my children have messed up badly, yes, I have been disappointed and have allowed them to experience the natural consequences of their disobedience. Yet I hope they will learn from their mistakes and change for the better. And my love for them remains forever fixed.

A Scientific Perspective

Most scientific evidence indicates that modern humans arose in Africa about 180,000 years ago. Interestingly, humans largely remained in a few distinct locations for almost 100,000 years. Archeological evidence from about 80,000 years ago, especially around burial sites of these populations, shows signs of abstract reasoning and the capacity of humans to differentiate themselves as individuals (all

System 2 characteristics). These social changes were mirrored by radical advances in technology and the great migration of populations throughout Africa and into Europe and Asia. These early humans also began to display proof that they were capable of deep love and relationships. For instance, they mourned the deaths of their loved ones by placing their most valuable possessions in the gravesites of the deceased.

The scientific evidence,[5] including a study from my own laboratory,[6] suggests that at this point in time, the human brain and particularly the neocortex dramatically increased in complexity and size. As a result, I believe, humans reached a much higher level of complexity that facilitated their capacity for System 2 reasoning and all that comes with it, including awareness of morality and the ability to examine and understand, override our basal System 1 survival instincts, love selflessly, and recognize *Self*.

No one knows for certain what caused this sudden increase in brain capacity. Much like the creation/Big Bang debate, scientists and theologians are likely to provide their own explanations. We do know, however, that the shift brought with it the human capacity to think, plan, form relationships, and work cooperatively in groups. On a more sobering note, I think this shift also made humans aware that they were separated from one another and would experience loneliness and ultimately death.

The Problem of Separateness

Make no mistake about it, at the center of our human condition is the desperate desire to escape the prison of our separateness. Most of us spend our lives trying to overcome loneliness through connections and relationships with others, in both healthy and unhealthy ways (more on this in chapter 9). With modern technological advancements, it is easy, at least on the surface, to connect with others. Just look at some of the overwhelming evidence.

- According to Pew research, 22 percent of adults ages twenty-five to thirty-four have used online dating, and its popularity among older singles is growing dramatically.[7]
- A staggering 91 percent of adults ages eighteen to thirty-four; 85 percent ages thirty-five to fifty-four; and 69 percent ages fifty-five and over use Facebook, with dramatic growth continuing on Instagram, Twitter, and Tumblr.[8]
- Sixty-four percent of Americans own a smartphone; 67 percent of these smartphone owners constantly check their phones for messages, alerts, or calls—even if they don't hear the phone ring or vibrate. Forty-four percent of owners keep their phones next to their beds at night so they don't miss any messages or calls as they sleep. Forty-six percent of owners describe their cell phones as "something they can't imagine living without."[9]

In our desperate attempt to avoid loneliness and insignificance, we spend incredible amounts of time connecting with others via social media. A recent study by *New York Times* bestselling authors Joseph Grenny and David Maxfield indicates that most of us craft a persona by posting status updates and photos that make our lives seem special and meaningful so others will be interested in us. In the process, however, we miss out on life's most important and enjoyable events.[10] In a recent poll reported in *The Telegraph*, one-third of those sampled admitted they felt lonely looking at their social media feeds.[11] It is ironic that our antidote to separateness can make us feel even more alone.

The Desperate Unrest Created by Our Awareness of Death

My father and I shared a close relationship. He meant the world to me. When Dad was alive, we talked on the phone almost every day. He was so proud of me and always told me (and anyone who would listen) so. I did not realize the finality of death until he died seventeen years ago. For months following his passing, I would call his telephone number just to listen to his voice on the answering machine. I particularly looked forward to hearing the ending of his message, a phrase he always used: "Have a blessed day." Then one day when I called, there was no voice mail. Someone had erased it, likely by accident. I cried for hours. Mourning his death, I was distraught by my separateness from my father. And no matter how much faith I have that I will see him again, I do not know how or when.

My father's passing did not just speak of my immense grief; it also reminded me that one day I, too, will die. I study a biological process called *apoptosis*, programmed cell death. Apoptosis tells scientists that every cell in our bodies has a specific life span, an expiration date. At that well-defined point in time, each cell initiates a program that facilitates its death in an orderly fashion. Death is built into the smallest units of our bodies. As a result, our bodies are genetically programmed to age and die. The day I was born, the clock began ticking.

Many questions surround the topic of mortality and dominate our feelings of separateness. When will I die? How?

What if my spouse or child dies before me? What happens after death? These questions linger and instill fear in our minds about the future, the unknown. It is important to note that being afraid of dying is natural, as is reflection of our knowledge of our own mortality.

To address this topic, it is necessary to pull back from my comfort zones of well-defined biological, philosophical, and psychological disciplines to the deep end of the pool where my personal faith and the mystical reside. As I said in the introduction, these are the big questions that stretch well beyond science's capacity to address them. However, even scientists are forced to move into these areas if they are to consider our human condition in this life and beyond.

As a Christian, I choose the path of faith in Jesus Christ and believe I will gain immortality through that relationship. Still, I understand that this life is full of mystery and questions and wonder. I love The Chronicles of Narnia and have read the seven books in the series to my four children. In the last paragraph of the final book in the series (*The Last Battle*), C. S. Lewis writes some of my favorite words:

> And for us this is the end of all the stories, and we can most truly say that they all lived happily ever after. But for them it was only the beginning of the real story. All their life in this world and all their adventures in Narnia had only been the cover and the title page: now at last they were beginning Chapter One of the Great Story which no one on earth has read: which goes on forever: in which every chapter is better than the one before.[12]

The human condition of separateness is the source of much of our inner unrest. We search for meaning. We seek to belong. We desire relationship. We long to cure our loneliness. We question the mysteries of the spiritual life. We come face-to-face with the looming shadow of death. All these things create in us a drive to find answers and alleviate our pain. I love what Mother Teresa reminded us: "The greatest disease in the West today is not TB or leprosy; it is being unwanted, unloved, and uncared for. We can cure physical diseases with medicine, but the only cure for loneliness, despair, and hopelessness is love."[13]

When Everything Seems Meaningless

Almost a decade ago and during a difficult period of my life, I took my first church mission trip to Africa with a team of twenty-five others. Partnering with the charitable organization Samaritan's Feet, our team traveled to eight locations around the Masoyi community in South Africa over the course of ten days, helping orphans affected by HIV/AIDS. At the time, this disease had wiped out a generation of young parents and orphaned twenty thousand children in that community alone. We helped bring food, water, shoes, and deworming medications to close to two thousand orphans during our visit.

Before leaving the States, I am almost embarrassed to admit that I had not given the trip much thought. I travel often, and while I had never been to Africa, I thought at a minimum the visit to this great continent was an item to check off my bucket list. My lack of introspection prior to the trip probably had to do with the intense pressure and anxiety I was under both at home and at work. I was depressed, lonely, empty. Nothing could alleviate or remove these deep inner feelings. Nothing mattered because, in the end, life seemed meaningless to me.

During this time, I found an alliance with King Solomon, deemed the wisest man who ever lived, and particularly with his opening words in Ecclesiastes, a book of wisdom in the Bible. As a scientist, I deeply respect this sacred writ for its honest recognition of the human condition. In the following passage, King Solomon presents an incredible System 2 analysis of what this means, and exactly where I was emotionally at the time.

> "Meaningless! Meaningless!"
>   says the Teacher.
> "Utterly meaningless!
>   Everything is meaningless."
> What do people gain from all their labors
>   at which they toil under the sun?
> Generations come and generations go,
>   but the earth remains forever.
> The sun rises and the sun sets,
>   and hurries back to where it rises. . . .
> What has been will be again,
>   what has been done will be done again;
>   there is nothing new under the sun. . . .
> No one remembers the former generations,
>   and even those yet to come
> will not be remembered
>   by those who follow them.
>   Ecclesiastes 1:2–5, 9, 11

The author's words are ripe with a fundamental restlessness and hopelessness. If we look at the evidence of our lives on the surface, nothing we do seems to matter. We live, we die, and we take nothing with us. The ceaseless cycles of nature

111

endure, but our existence on this planet does not. If we are lucky, a generation from now, few at most will remember we were once alive.

Reading King Solomon's cry of despair further charged my feelings of insignificance and loneliness, despite how blessed I was and grateful for my family and burgeoning career.

About to Be Messed Up!

After thirty long hours of travel, our team finally touched down at the international airport in Johannesburg, where we boarded a school bus for the final six-hour leg to our destination, a small Bible college surrounded by a huge barbed wire fence in the middle of a large shantytown. Following a few hours of sleep, we were welcomed with a hearty breakfast and a devotional by Manny Ohome, a large African man with a big smile. Manny was originally from Nigeria, had moved to the United States to play college basketball, became a very successful businessman, and now was president of Samaritan's Feet.

Though I can't remember what the devotional was about, I will never forget what this man said to me right after he closed in prayer. We had not yet been formally introduced, but for reasons I did not understand at the time, he picked me out of the crowd and walked straight toward me. Looking me square in the eyes, Manny said, "God told me that you are about to be messed up!"

Taken aback, I stared back at him as if he were crazy. I didn't know what he meant by his bold statement. Who did he think he was? Not knowing what to say in response, I simply nodded my head.

Our team's first task was to provide shoes for hundreds of beautiful children ages two to eighteen. They gathered in a long line and for hours waited while our team washed the feet of each child and put a pair of clean shoes on them. For many, it was their first pair. I had the privilege of praying with the orphans after they received their shoes. Many of them recounted brief though heartbreaking stories of unthinkable suffering and abuse when I asked how I could pray for them. I felt helpless, uttering what felt like trite words in the midst of their devastating lives. What good would a pair of shoes and a prayer really do?

Two days later, Manny's prophetic words became reality. Our group traveled to a banana plantation. I cannot explain what happened the moment I stepped off the bus and my feet touched down on the red African soil, but I immediately sensed my life would forever be changed at this time and by this place.

As I turned my head to scan the landscape, my eyes first fell on the hundreds of children confined behind a tangled and rusty barbed wire fence. The older ones stuck their heads through the sharp coils to get a better look at the "rich" Americans walking toward them. I noticed off to the side a group of about fifty infants, likely two years old and under, sitting in muddy sewer water. Some were playing, splashing about in the mosquito-infested puddle. But most were crying, wailing at the top of their lungs.

I was inexplicably drawn to one particular child who appeared to be about two years of age. His eyes were deep yellow from liver failure as a result of AIDS and tuberculosis, his face badly distorted from a birth defect and the ravages of malnutrition. He was crying, but only halfheartedly, as he had cried for so long without anyone paying attention. I asked one of the "grannies," the older women in charge of the smaller kids, the name of this child. She shook her head and shrugged. She didn't know. And that is when I realized none of the children behind the barbed wire had a name. This took my breath away.

Staring at the tearful baby, my instinct was to scoop him up in my arms. But as we locked eyes, I thought with fear, "I can't hold him. It's too much of a risk." As a biomedical researcher, I knew the ramifications of contracting a drug-resistant strain of tuberculosis.

In that moment, for the first time in my life, I heard God speak to my heart. Let me say that up to that point I had always been the one in the crowd who scoffed with scientific arrogance whenever I would hear someone say they heard the voice of God. But standing there, staring at a malnourished, crying baby in the sweltering African heat, I felt in my heart as clear as day God asking me, "Who are you?" And then, "Whose are you?"

I believe the first question was not an inquiry of my identity. I assume God knows exactly who I am. I believe it was a reminder of my humanity. I was connected to this child through the family of the human race in ways I did not comprehend. And in showing love to this child and others roaming around the banana plantation, I was showing love to the entire human race, including my *Self*. This understanding was well beyond my primitive System 1, which is capable of caring only about my *Self* and my family. It came from the powerful System 2 and its connection to God and the universe.

The question "Whose are you?" prompted me to realize that I, like this crying child, was a child of God. And though

I had been living in a spiritual world that was oblivious to me most of the time, the present moment challenged me to step up to a life of faith beyond mere words, theology, and religious tradition. Because I was in a personal relationship with God, I had a responsibility to be his arms, his feet, his love in this and every situation following.

I immediately picked up the child from the muddy water, wiped his face with my shirt, and pressed his face against mine. Holding his emaciated body tight, I softly sang the same lullaby my mom had sung to me. "Bye oh baby, oh bye, oh baby." Almost immediately, the little guy stopped crying. He looked right into my eyes, and for the first and only time in my life, I saw the face of God.

This moment changed everything. My perception of the human condition and my role on this planet shifted. My perspective that everything was meaningless dissipated, and a new one of purpose was created. My dear African brother Manny was right. I was "messed up"—messed up in the most meaningful way possible that would forever change the trajectory of my life.

The Power of Love

Why was this moment so powerful? What was it about that one particular child in a sea of starving, impoverished, and diseased children that forever transformed my heart? How did Manny know I was going to get messed up on this banana plantation?

I don't know for certain the answers to these questions, and I suspect I never will in this life. Perhaps you can relate. Maybe you, too, experienced an inexplicable event that moved you toward lasting change. While we may never grasp the full meaning of these mystical and dynamic occurrences, what matters is that they influence and, most importantly, reshape us.

While it has taken me almost a decade to grasp, I believe the African experience put me on a pathway to begin to make sense of my existence. On that day in the banana plantation, I began to realize that life is much simpler than I had ever imagined. I have only one job during my time on this planet: to love. This, like the human condition, is a first principle. If you start each day with the intention of loving, everything else in your life (your relationships, your career, your mortality, all your efforts, how you spend your time) will take care of itself. And together they will result in a beautiful, meaningful, and joyful life. Just as Mother Teresa said, love is the cure to our loneliness, despair, and hopelessness.

I also began to comprehend the paradoxical nature of giving. A common myth about giving—whether our time, our money, our energy, or our effort—is that giving something means giving up something else. In this perspective, giving is not a sustainable resource. The more you give, the more you will drain your reservoir.

Individuals who are focused on overcoming their isolation by dominating or being dominated have a market approach to giving. They are willing to give only if they get something in return. These people will donate a thousand dollars to a charitable organization so they can be recognized for their efforts on a stage or in an ad. They will sacrifice a weekend to help a friend on the silent condition that this person "owes them one."

People who give to receive typically believe that giving is a sacrifice. They suffer or are certainly inconvenienced by sending that check, volunteering time after work, or taking that mission trip. And if they don't see any get for their give, they feel cheated. I see this frequently in churches where giving is almost portrayed as an act of martyrdom, as if we should do it for that reason as opposed to experiencing joy.

My experience in Africa turned this convoluted concept on its head. It provided me with a new economy of love. There was only one solution, one antidote to our human condition of separateness: to love others, and not because others will give back but because the universe and its Creator will return the *Self*-less act in ways beyond our imagination.

Being surrounded by thousands of orphans and being blessed to have the opportunity to serve Christ through them channeled into my life incredible love, joy, meaning, and power. In fact, merely by giving my *Self*, I rediscovered my life and found my *Self*, who I was meant to be. About once a week I wear a T-shirt to work that reads, "I need Africa more than Africa needs me." I am convinced that, if not for that first trip to this special continent, I could have lost my *Self*, my purpose for living, forever.

Even now, I don't claim to have the answers to the central issues of our human condition. However, I am certain that our understanding of and how we respond to these first principles determines everything about the quality of life we will live.

Reflection: The Pathway to Rewire Your Mind

1. Have you ever felt alone? Have you ever thought life or your actions were meaningless? How did you respond to these feelings?

2. How does modern society contribute to feelings of isolation or insignificance?

3. Have you experienced the death of a loved one? How did you reflect on the finality?

4. Where or how do you find meaning in your life? What gives you purpose?

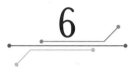

6

Right and Wrong Matters

For as he thinks in his heart, so is he.

Proverbs 23:7 NKJV

My friend John grew up in the late 1960s in the backwoods of South Carolina, where racism reigned. In fact, one of his uncles and a few parents of some of his friends from school were members of the KKK. The poison of racism was deeply embedded in John's environment through family, misguided societal norms, and pressure from his peers.

John was in the first grade when legal segregation ended. He vividly remembers the fear in the eyes of the little black girls and boys who became his new classmates. He also remembers the hate spewed toward these children and how it seemed almost everyone around him urged him to treat these African American children as bad, even evil.

And yet, deep in his heart, John knew something wasn't right. He liked his new friends. Even in the midst of every influence to follow the crowd and treat these new students poorly, hurling degrading insults their way, he could not ignore the gnawing thought that this behavior was wrong. So despite constant violent intimidation and threats from others, even from his own family members, John treated all of the new students with the kindness and compassion they deserved. He walked beside them in the halls. He talked to them when they were scared. He sat next to them when no one else would.

What made John refuse to submit to the clamoring voices of racism all around him? Why did he choose diversity and love over bigotry and hate? Why did he choose to take a stand and be persecuted when the easiest thing in the world would have been to go along with the crowd? What gave John a clear picture of morality under circumstances in which most everyone else got it so wrong?

Along with first principles, morality sets in motion the next several chapters on reframing the different aspects of our lives for one reason: this key component of being human is the foundation on which everything else stands. It will be impossible to put the rest of your life in order until you establish consistent moral principles. In order to grow as individuals and as a society at large, we need to calibrate our moral compasses. We must become men and women who long for truth and meaning, who seek to do the right thing no matter the cost. Abolitionist Henry Ward Beecher said, "A man that has lost moral sense is like a man in battle with both of his legs shot off: he has nothing to stand on."[1]

In realizing the importance of morality, I spent the past two years intensely studying how it is developed and its relationship to free will. Much of this time was spent in discussions with my colleague Kevin Jung, a brilliant philosopher and associate professor of Christian ethics at Wake Forest University. In chapter 4, I introduced a model of moral development that I have based on this research. This chapter will highlight my key findings regarding its relevance to our lives and particularly our futures.

Key Components of Morality

The Source of Morality

I love the opening line of Crosby, Stills, Nash & Young's 1970s classic "Teach Your Children Well": "You, who are on the road, must have a code that you can live by." Philosophers and theologians have both argued that humans have a natural understanding or intuitive sense of morality, the difference between right and wrong. I call this the *moral knowledge condition*.

Both C. S. Lewis in his classic *Mere Christianity* and leading New Testament scholar N. T. Wright in *Simply Christian* broaden this idea by pointing out that the existence of this instinctive knowledge is evidence that a supernatural force, namely God, created a basic instinctual moral code for humankind. The observation of a moral code across a wide variety of cultures was a major reason Lewis, a former atheist, shifted his worldview to theism.

Wright says:

Get rid of "God," and you no longer have a "problem of evil." All you have is unwelcome "attitudes" or "prejudices."

Not that people can easily live like that. They quickly invent new "moralities" around the one or two fixed points that appear to transcend that subjective, emotive analysis: the badness of Adolf Hitler, the goodness of ecological activism, the importance of "embracing the Other," and so on. Better than nothing, perhaps; but people who try to sail the moral seas with that equipment look suspiciously like a handful of survivors clinging to a broken spar as the ship goes down and the sharks close in.[2]

I, too, believe God is the source of this moral compass. And in the absence of severe mental illness or abuse, this yardstick of good and evil, right and wrong, what is fair and what is unjust, is present in all of us.

However, I have found that aligning our inner principles with God's moral laws, the instinctual set of virtues that spur our convictions, will often place us in the minority. But this is what Christ instructed us to do. He said, "Enter through the narrow gate. For wide is the gate and broad is the road that leads to destruction, and many enter through it. But small is the gate and narrow the road that leads to life, and only a few find it" (Matt. 7:13–14). It is much easier to approach morally challenging situations by adhering to our thoughtless, default response of primitive System 1, like being suspicious of those who look or act different from us or turning a blind eye to someone in need. John took a stance against the racial mistreatment of his peers and paid the heavy price of being ostracized and persecuted for it. The pathway of morality is narrow indeed.

As difficult as it may be at times, living grounded in love as a man or a woman of moral integrity is what leads to peace, joy, and purpose. God's message to "love your neighbor as yourself" (Mark 12:31), for instance, is a life-sustaining approach because of its natural reciprocal nature. Somehow and in many ways, the love you give away comes back manifold. You learned this in the previous chapter.

I believe John's story makes a great case for a human intuition of fairness, justice, and right and wrong. As a Christian, I am saddened by the positions many Southern churches I attended during this critical moment in history chose to take. At best, they were silent on the subject of racism. At worst, in support of their prejudiced positions, they used the same Bible and in many cases the same verses as those who fought for civil rights. Consequently, the church did not provide direction or support for God's moral law for people like John. And that meant being in opposition to the one organization that should have been the first to exemplify what it means to love our neighbor.

Moral Development

Why did John have the capacity to make such courageous moral choices in such a difficult situation? I am not sure I will ever know the complete answer to this extraordinarily complex question. I do believe, however, that over time his choices and experiences nurtured his intrinsic moral knowledge, which developed into his high-level morality.

Consistent with our understanding of brain plasticity, the process of moral development begins in early childhood and involves making often difficult System 2 choices centered on God's natural laws. Like our thoughts, our moral choices eventually become habits and automatic reactions. By choosing to act in accordance with our moral knowledge condition and not the self-preservation of System 1 instincts and needs, we alter our brain DNA. This, in turn, orchestrates brain wiring that aligns with God-designed morality. Repeating these choices consistently over time strengthens this wiring and makes it even more powerful. In the same manner, when we make immoral choices, we wire our brains in a way that enhances our likelihood of repeating the same unprincipled actions in the future.

I call this unconscious remembering of our past responses to morally challenging situations and its effect on future choices *moral memory*. Moral memory ensures that over time we form our own morality. Eventually, how we act and respond according to our moral compass becomes our character, thereby locking in that moral memory. Once this happens, it becomes much easier to resolve morally difficult situations because our responses become automatic. We react in positive and meaningful ways or negative and selfish ways without thinking, depending on our past choices. We have wired our morality.

Like other critical aspects of our personality, our morality is also highly affected by our early childhood environment. Think back to the relationships you had growing up with your mother and/or father and significant adults. How did they help (or not) build moral fibers into your being? Did they practice what they preached? Did they do the right thing when no one was looking? Did they advocate for human equality? Were they compassionate toward those in pain and the less fortunate? Did they tell lies to get ahead? Did they talk about others behind their backs?

One of the most important events in John's life was watching his mother's reaction to a group of family members and friends who spoke of how none of their children, nor any white kid for that matter, would attend school on the first day of desegregation. This petite five-foot-two woman passionately lectured this ignorant crowd from the basis of Jesus's teachings. She reminded them they went to church every Sunday and challenged them to think about the cruel and insensitive things they were saying in light of the Bible they claimed to believe in. She prompted them to think about how those new kids were children, human beings, who feared for their very lives. John was especially moved when his mother told these people, "You better believe my son will not only stand with these kids but also even hold their hands if that will make them feel safer and more loved."

This was 1964. Teach your children well.

Moral Responsibility

Philosophers spend a great deal of time addressing the issue of free will in the context of personal responsibility, especially as it relates to morality. A key theme of these philosophical discussions is whether it is fair or just to hold a person accountable for a morally wrong decision if they had no other choice.

Free will, or the principle of alternative possibilities, means that a person is "morally responsible for what he has done only if he could have done otherwise."[3] As I have previously mentioned, determinists believe that no one is responsible for their actions because all actions result from antecedent physical causes, which result from previous actions. This camp would accept phrases such as "I couldn't help it" or "I had no choice" as completely valid defenses in any given morally questionable situation.

I believe otherwise. As I have written, individuals who make free System 2 choices in morally challenging situations change their DNA, wire their brains in a particular manner, and ensure their subsequent responses will be more consistent with their initial System 2 choices. Collectively, all these choices over time become habits that ultimately form their character. Now, because these individuals were responsible for their initial choices, they are ultimately responsible for their character.

So is there ever a time when we can legitimately deny responsibility for our actions? A critical question that often arises among psychologists and within our legal system is whether children who have had intense and long-term exposure to toxic environments can be held responsible for their actions as adults. Can a boy whose father forced him at age eleven to have sex with a prostitute and, consequently, learned from his dad how to objectify and degrade women for his pleasure be held accountable for participating in sex trafficking as an adult? What about the little girl who grew up with a violent, alcoholic mother who was also emotionally and physically abusive? Can she be held accountable for bullying others in high school? What extent of responsibility should these individuals own when their brain circuitry and resulting destructive emotional dysfunctions developed from their toxic environments?

Indeed, it has long been recognized that early exposure to severe forms of stress, abuse, and neglect is a significant risk factor for the development of subsequent psychopathology, including severe anxiety disorders, post-traumatic stress disorder, depression, bipolar disorder, and schizophrenia.[4] That said, I believe the answer depends on whether the

extent of the toxic exposure induced psychological damage and, consequently, whether the damage is permanent
or modifiable.

This brings to mind Shin Dong-hyuk, whose horrific
journey was captured in his biography, *Escape from Camp
14*. Shin was born in a slave labor camp in North Korea in
1982 and escaped in 2005. For over twenty-three years, Shin
witnessed prisoners, including women and children, being
tortured for trivial acts such as hiding food; the deaths of
thousands from starvation; and the public executions of
dozens every year. Part of Shin's own finger was mutilated
as punishment for accidently dropping a sewing machine.
Beginning at birth, Shin learned to survive by any means,
including reporting the activities of fellow innocent inmates
to the camp guards for reward.

Shin admitted with great shame that he had played a
decisive role in the execution of his mother and brother.
When he was around fifteen years old, he overheard the
two planning an escape and ratted them out to the guards.
Both subsequently were tortured, and then his mother was
hanged and his brother shot. In a blog posted on his bi-
ographer Blaine Harden's website, Shin admitted, "I was
jealous of my brother because my mother liked him more
than me. My mother never liked me much. She beat me
much more than my brother. She never paid attention to
my birthday."[5]

At the time, Shin believed both his mother and his brother
deserved to die and even felt some level of satisfaction watching their execution. Clearly, this young man endured such a
dehumanizing and baneful upbringing that his moral knowledge condition was gravely distorted. On many fronts, Shin

was born a victim. His brain architecture developed in an environment that rewarded evil, encouraged apathy and a lack of remorse, and normalized torture and degradation of humans. Was this young man any more responsible for his brain development than a Hiroshima survivor is at fault for getting cancer as a result of their exposure to radiation? I don't believe so.

Let's consider a less extreme hypothetical example. Joe and Jack are two brothers who grew up under difficult and stressful circumstances. Their father abused prescription drugs, and their mother was verbally abusive. Though tragic, their upbringing was not catastrophic enough to destroy their capacity to recognize God's moral laws within them. Therefore, by the time they reach adulthood, they have some ability to experience System 2 deliberation in morally challenging situations.

Unfortunately, because of their tumultuous past, both Joe and Jack engage in unhealthy behaviors that cause considerable destruction to themselves and others. Joe likes his vodka too much and has serious control issues, often dominating women in relationships. Jack exhibits narcissistic behavior and always puts his needs and wants before others, perpetuating a cycle of broken relationships and loneliness. Because they still more or less accurately sense their moral knowledge condition, both Joe and Jack recognize that they are responsible for their wrong behavioral patterns and that the path they are on will likely lead to a grim future. They know they need help.

In their early forties, both brothers separately see a therapist once a week in hopes of feeling better. The counselor does a wonderful job helping both men recognize the impact of their early negative environments on their actions as adults and the reasons for their inability to make choices consistent with their moral knowledge condition. Both men learn tools for utilizing System 2 reasoning to override their System 1 responses when faced with triggers from childhood.

At this point, while Joe and Jack, like us all, may be influenced by their past to some degree, each has reappraised it and is able to utilize his System 2 freedom to form new responses to morally challenging situations. That said, Joe may choose to ignore his moral knowledge condition and continue to take advantage of others. Is he now responsible for his present character and future actions as a result? I believe the answer is yes. Because he at least partially rewired his mind, Joe is capable of System 2 reasoning, and his present and future choices are no longer under the control of his past. Joe has the capacity to do otherwise and is thus responsible for how he chooses to act.

And what of Shin? After intense cognitive behavioral therapy, he has come far emotionally and mentally. Today he works for Liberty in North Korea (LiNK), a nonprofit organization that raises awareness of human rights issues and helps refugees in that country. On December 2, 2012, Shin was featured on *60 Minutes*. In that interview, he remarked, "When I see videos of the Holocaust it moves me to tears. I think I am still evolving—from an animal to a human."[6] Clearly, Shin has recovered his inherent moral knowledge condition and is now profoundly impacted by moral atrocities such as genocide.

One of the most surprising and powerful aspects of humans in general and of the human brain in particular is their incredible resiliency. Despite how we were raised or the horrors of our teenage or young adult lives, change is possible.

We can alter our capacity to make better moral decisions that correspond with God's will for our lives. And no matter what our past influences and environments, we will always be in future situations with opportunities to do the right thing.

Rationalization: Morality's Slippery Slope

When we face morally challenging situations, we do one of three things. One, we respond in a manner consistent with God's moral laws, as John did. Two, we unconsciously act against God's morality. And three, we choose to do the wrong thing and justify these decisions with excuses. I will focus on this latter very popular response.

Many people respond to morally challenging situations by minimizing their capacity to act or their own individual responsibility. We come up with a slew of excuses not to exact God's moral principles just so we can feel better about our decisions.

A few years ago, a photo appeared on the front page of the *New York Post* that generated a widespread public outcry. It showed a man who had been pushed into a subway well and was desperately trying to escape seconds before an oncoming subway crushed and killed him. Questions immediately arose as to why the photographer chose to take a picture rather than help the man get out. The photographer stated in an interview that he was not "strong enough to physically lift the victim himself"[7] and opted to use his camera to continually flash at and alert the subway driver. Though I cannot be certain of this man's genuine intentions, I believe when he came face-to-face with a morally challenging situation, he rationalized the importance or the need for his role in the event.

In the same vein, there is a human response known as the *bystander effect* or *bystander apathy*, which diffuses an individual's moral responsibility in a crowd. The principle was popularized following the 1964 murder of Kitty Genovese in Kew Gardens, New York. Genovese was stabbed to death outside her apartment while others watched and did not step in to assist or even call the police. In fact, it is interesting, sad, and predictable that the probability of an individual getting help in a traumatic situation is inversely related to the number of bystanders watching it. The more people present, the less likely someone will step in.

In an age of greater and greater entitlement mentalities and moral relativism, I believe our excuses may pose one of the greatest threats to the fabric of modern society. What is so scary is that the more we use excuses to justify moral inaction or unethical behavior, the more we truly believe our own lies and thereby provide avenues to skirt our moral responsibility.

Ethics Alarms, a popular ethics-focused website, recently published a list of twenty-four common unethical rationalizations people use to not do the right thing. They include:

- "Everybody does it."
- No harm, no foul.
- It's just business.
- Do it to them before they do it to you.
- Just this one time.
- What I did was fine because it all worked out for the best.
- "If I don't do it, somebody else will."[8]

Like moral memory, unethical rationalization will become our predominant System 1 habit if we consistently validate our choices with excuses. This is why it is important to empha-size why and how to choose right over wrong. *Self*-awareness about how our own feelings and behaviors follow our thoughts (and excuses) is critical to our moral development. Christ emphasized this philosophy in his teaching. In Scripture, he appeared most troubled by those who focused on judging others before reflecting on their own conduct. He had some harsh words for these people. "You hypocrite, first take the plank out of your own eye, and then you will see clearly to remove the speck from your brother's eye" (Matt. 7:5).

A few years ago, a childhood friend called and asked to sit down and talk over coffee. I could hear a sense of desperation in her voice. When we met, she looked visibly concerned, though I hadn't the faintest clue why. As we waited for our lattes, she looked me point-blank in the eyes and said, "I'm leaving my husband."

I knew this couple well, as her husband was also a child-hood friend, so I was stunned. "Why?" I asked.

Still reeling from shock, I listened as my friend rattled off a list of reasons. He was having an emotional affair with a co-worker; she had not been sexually satisfied for years; he acted distant toward her; she was "kind of" seeing someone else; her husband was always busy working; and, bottom line, he'd be better off without her. I remember how astonished I was to hear her list her rationalizations and nonchalantly slip in the critical, morally relevant fact that she was having an affair. I knew my friend's husband was a good man who deeply loved his wife. He would have been willing to see a therapist to work through any of the problems. I also was aware that my friend had some deep childhood abuse issues that she had never addressed, and I believed they influenced her current thinking in ways she couldn't imagine. Please understand I wasn't judgmental of her actions. I was deeply concerned that she was making a huge mistake.

I ended our conversation by saying, "I will always love you like a sister, but please do yourself a huge favor before you make this tragic decision. Be honest with yourself. If you continue to see the guy on the side and choose to end your current marriage, do it with honesty. Admit that your secret affair will cause great damage to both you and your family. Your life and legacy as a wife and mother are on the line here. Respect yourself and your husband enough to do what you feel you must do at least in truth."

Any excuse that you use as a reason to do wrong things or to lie wires your mind to the point where the untruths become a System 1 habit that blocks you from realizing the consequences of your immoral actions. In time, your character will be based on your chronic distortions of truth.

We human beings are not naturally great at judging our own feelings and behaviors. Without deep introspection, prayer, a support network of wise and trusted friends and family, and/or a spiritual community, we remain limited by our own realities and thus can justify or make sense of any wrongful action. Without truth, we unconsciously create a fabricated existence that will ultimately destroy our capacity to sense our moral knowledge condition and cause us to live in the absence of meaning and significance.

Morality Breeds Positive Changes

As I write this chapter, I am sitting in a hotel room in Myrtle Beach, South Carolina. I think the reason I am here this weekend is to remind myself just how far we have come as a nation since John's time. This morning I took a stroll down the boardwalk, reveling in the colorful tapestry of diversity everywhere I looked. Adorable little kids of many ethnicities laughed and played with one another. Couples of different races held hands. While our society has certainly not solved all of the problems surrounding racial discrimination and human equality, we have made tremendous strides toward a better future for our children and their progeny.

We owe it to our *Selves* to be vulnerable and painfully honest, to quit defending and rationalizing our System 1 feelings and responses based on selfishness and fear rather than love. We must learn to be accountable for our actions whether good or bad. We must take responsibility for our choices and understand the role they play in our future.

Take some time before you read the next chapter to assess your moral compass by answering the following questions. Your responses will be pivotal in how you react to the remainder of this book. Once you have a clear understanding of your morality, it will be easier for you to understand and overcome the struggles you face in regard to tragedy, raising kids, relationships, intimacy, and sexuality.

Reflection: The Pathway to Rewire Your Mind

1. From where do you get your standards of morality? By what natural laws or philosophy do you orient your moral compass?

2. What do you believe are your greatest morality blind spots? Can you remember a time when you got it right? And another when you got it wrong?

3. How much time and energy do you focus toward your *Self* and your own family as opposed to looking outward and loving and helping others? Have you found a healthy balance?

4. What do you believe is your most-used excuse for not doing the right thing? What does this say about you?

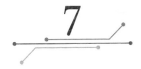

7

When Tragedy Strikes

The God I believe in doesn't send us the problem;
He gives us the strength to cope with the problem.

Rabbi Harold Kushner, *When Bad Things
Happen to Good People*

Years ago, a good friend of mine became pregnant. Like
most mothers, she was elated. She was proud of her changing
body, excited about planning the nursery and buying cute
baby things, and daydreamed of all the things she would do
with her little one. A few months into her pregnancy, she
underwent a genetic test. The result was shocking. The baby
was diagnosed with a severe genetic abnormality.

A few years after the baby was born, my friend confided in
me. While she shared how her child was nothing less than a
blessing and she couldn't imagine her life any different, she also
admitted feeling disappointed when she first heard the news.

My friend offered a telling analogy based on something she had read.[1] She said that in becoming pregnant, it was as if she was headed to Paris to live the rest of her life in a beautiful villa surrounded by lavender and olive orchards. She learned to speak French fluently. And after double-checking her packing list, she boarded a plane, excited to experience this new adventure and new life.

However, the flight seemed to take much longer than scheduled. After the plane touched down, she walked down the Jetway into an unfamiliar setting. No one spoke French. The airport signs were in a different language. Even the people looked different. She quickly realized she had landed in a strange city that was anything but Paris. No one could explain why her flight had not reached its intended destination. And no one was able to correct the problem. With no way out, my friend was stuck in a new place, alone and feeling frightened, abandoned, and betrayed.

While so far I have largely focused on exaggerated System 1 emotions and reactions, our System 1 instincts and drives also interact with System 2 to create powerful visions of our future. Childhood dreams often become adult aspirations. My friend had a very successful career, but she also wanted a family. Like most little girls, she had always dreamed of becoming a mother. There is overwhelming scientific evidence that early memories create circuitry in System 1 brain regions. Once these visions with their fairy-tale endings are set in our minds, they are incredibly difficult to alter. My friend's early childhood experiences and dreams gave rise to brain wiring that powerfully shaped a narrative and a desire for a family in her future.

As we approach adulthood, we begin to understand that uncertainty and pain abound. Our plans, our hopes, our dreams, and our world can change on a dime. This happens when a spouse or a child is diagnosed with a terminal illness, when we have to care for an elderly parent diagnosed with Alzheimer's, when we lose our job and can't make ends meet, when we receive a cancer diagnosis, when the dream we worked so hard to attain is crushed, when our spouse walks away from the marriage. The list goes on and on.

It is shocking to be struck by life events that cause severe pain, suffering, and stress. We can't believe this is happening to us. We wonder what we did wrong. We question the goodness and even the existence of God. Much of this pain also stems from the expectations that were wired in the System 1 regions of our minds much earlier in life. This often is where many of us get stuck. And this is where we must utilize System 2 to surrender these early dreams, connect with God and our strengths, and reframe our lives.

The Fundamentals of Reframing Tragedy

Reframing loss, illness, or grief is a journey from exile. Consciously and unconsciously, we feel tremendous anger, despair, depression, and resentment. Waves of emotion overwhelm our minds. Reframing is not about minimizing, fighting, or ignoring what we have been through; it is about returning from a destination where we feel displaced, disconnected, or depressed. Although we cannot change what happened, we can change our thoughts, our perspective, and our approach to move forward in life.

While this chapter does not offer a step-by-step how-to plan to get over a tragic situation, it aims to show how you can get unstuck when you reflect on your experience and how to remove some roadblocks that can hinder the reframing process. If you currently have difficulty coping—if you are having trouble sleeping, feeling depressed and/or an overwhelming sense of hopelessness, abusing substances like alcohol or drugs, or suffering from debilitating nightmares or anxiety—I encourage you to seek help. Find a licensed counselor. Reach out to loved ones. Join a support group. You do not have to suffer alone.

Come to Peace with Your Beliefs about the Cause(s) of Tragedy

I am always blown away by the foolish things people say to someone going through heartbreak or tragedy. A few years ago, I attended a funeral service of a teenager who had committed suicide. As I stood in line waiting to speak with his parents, I struggled with what to say. Words did not come easily. I knew spouting a monologue or offering advice would be pointless. So I just told this couple who had endured an unthinkable loss how sorry I was and then hugged them tight. What else was there to say?

Unfortunately, I have heard perhaps well-intentioned but misguided people respond in these circumstances with phrases and clichés that only enhance the sufferer's pain or spotlight a disturbing theological perspective.

If your husband has left you for another woman, if your child has a fatal disease and is in the hospital for the tenth time, if you are dealing with a debilitating physical or mental illness, the last thing you want or need to hear is:

"This is God's will, and you have to accept it."
"God never gives us more than we can handle."

"God has selected you for this burden because he knows how strong you are."

Perhaps one of the most horrible statements I have heard was when someone approached a couple who had just suffered the loss of their only child. This person said, "I'm sorry you're sad. But God obviously needed your baby as an angel in heaven more than you did." I can say with confidence that was not, nor ever will be, the case.

In his book *The Will of God*, English theologian Leslie Weatherhead tells the profound story of being in India with a friend who had lost his young son in a cholera epidemic. Weatherhead walked beside his friend, who paced up and down the veranda of his home only a few feet away from his sleeping daughter, his only surviving child. The bereaved man turned to the great theologian and said, "Well, padre, it is the will of God. That's all there is to it. It is the will of God."[2]

Weatherhead gently disagreed. He loved his friend and knew him well enough to reply with the following words: "Suppose someone crept up the steps of the veranda tonight, while you all slept, and deliberately put a wad of cotton soaked in cholera germ culture over the little girl's mouth as she lay in that cot on the veranda, what would you think about that?"[3] The father was horrified and replied by saying he would kill the intruder and then asked why he would even suggest such a cruel thing.

Weatherhead quietly explained to his friend that that was what he had done when he had characterized his son's death as God's will. "Call your little boy's death the result of mass ignorance, call it mass folly, call it mass sin, if you like, call it bad drains or communal carelessness, but don't call it the will of God."[4]

What you attribute your tragedy to will make a huge difference in your capacity to reframe it. Whatever you have been through or are going through as you read these words, do not blame God for your suffering. Pin it on the uncertainty of the universe, the evil nature of humankind, or the freedom that God gave human beings to choose how to live and what to do, but not on God.

The tension of determining the source or cause of suffering is illustrated well in the biblical book of Job. While a complete thesis on this story is well beyond the scope of this book, I offer a brief overview.

Job is an incredibly fortunate, wealthy, and, above all else, godly man. One day Satan approaches God and proposes that the only reason Job is faithful is because of all the blessings God has graciously given him. To paraphrase the text, "He's a puppet on a string," Satan accuses. "Take all the good stuff away and then see what a respectable man of faith he really is" (see Job 1:9–11).

Confident in his servant's character, God puts Satan to the test and allows him to take and destroy all that Job has. In a series of tragic events, with not much pause in between, Satan destroys the man's livestock, kills all of his children and his servants, and afflicts him with painful sores all over his body. Understandably depressed and unable to make sense of the senseless, Job offers prayers peppered with questions and doubt. Yet he does not curse God. He remains faithful even when his cantankerous wife tries her best to convince her husband that the Almighty is at fault and undeserving of his unbending loyalty.

Job's three friends aren't much help. They suffer from incorrect assumptions resulting from bad theology. Unable to live with the mysteries of suffering, these three men have conversation after conversation with Job that circle back to their same theory: bad things happen to bad people, so Job must have done something wrong. The poor guy refuses to accept their hypothesis yet remains in a state of tension, not sure what to make of the God he serves. Toward the end of this story, God appears in a windstorm. While he does not provide an answer for Job's suffering, he makes it crystal clear that understanding issues this complex is well beyond human comprehension. God then rebukes Job's friends for their ignorance and gives Job a new future.

Outside of blaming God for orchestrating tragic events, some people of faith, whether traditional or otherwise, also ascribe guilt to the suffering party, calling it justice, karma, fate, or destiny. Some people even blame themselves for unexplainable incidents. There appears to be a strong need in humans to believe that we get what we deserve here on earth, even though there is evidence to the contrary all around us.

While I was writing this chapter, an earthquake struck Nepal, India, killing eight thousand people and injuring nineteen thousand. Were these twenty-seven thousand people evil and thus deserving to die or be hurt? Did all eleven million victims of the Holocaust cause their demise through selfish or greedy living? Do the children who lie bedridden in pediatric intensive care units in hospitals all over the world somehow warrant their misery and pain?

As I have said throughout this book, God seems to place an extraordinarily high emphasis on freedom. This is evidenced in nature, through the beauty of sunsets and the violence of hurricanes. This is evidenced in biology, through the body's ability to heal itself in an orderly fashion or mount a massive inflammatory response in the coronary artery that leads to a heart attack and death. And this is evidenced in human beings, through our freedom to do the right thing and make critical System 2 choices during our most difficult moments or reject God's love and compassion and live life our own way.

Get Real with Your Tragedy

Swiss psychiatrist Elisabeth Kübler-Ross introduced the idea of the five stages of grief in her 1969 book *On Death and Dying*. They include:

1. denial and isolation,
2. anger,
3. bargaining,
4. depression, and
5. acceptance.

Sadly, not everyone reaches the final stage of acceptance. Some tragedies are so sudden, unexpected, and disastrous that we never move past the first four stages. Our minds get stuck in System 1, replaying the same memories from the past over and over. When we are imprisoned in emotional overdrive by denial, isolation, anger, and resentment, playing "if only" scenarios in our heads, we cannot reframe our trauma and, consequently, rewire our minds.

I vividly remember a therapy session I had after a series of heartbreaking crises, one of which I will talk about in the next few pages. I was in complete denial of just how difficult my situation was. I told my counselor, "Oh sure, my situation stinks, but there are plenty of people, innocent children even, all over the world who have it much worse." I said (and thought) this a lot, not just during my therapy sessions. Since others could handle worse traumas than mine, I figured I should be able to be strong and control my own pain.

Having heard me repeat this statement numerous times, my therapist leaned toward me in his seat and looked deep into my sleep-deprived eyes. "Ski," he began, "you need to understand one thing: your life is horrible at this point in time. You have lost a marriage and a business and experienced a devastating loss. Those around you are falling apart with unthinkable pain. When you can begin to acknowledge these tragedies and their impact for what they are and release your emotions from that fortified prison in your mind, you might have a chance to dig out of this hole and come out on the other side. Otherwise, you are wasting both my time and yours."

Though his words stung, I appreciated his honesty. More importantly, I took his advice to heart. Mentally drained, I drove home from his office and finally realized I had to get real. I had to get honest with my situation, focus on my *Self*, and lean into God. And then, and only from that place of transparency, would I be able to begin to rebuild.

So how does one face reality and accept the pain of losing a loved one, receiving a terminal diagnosis, recovering from an addiction, getting served an eviction notice or divorce papers? I am not a therapist, so I can only speak from personal experience. Understand that the actual steps to reframing your tragedy or trauma will begin when you seek outside help and work through your deep issues with a counselor, professional spiritual advisor, mentor, or support group. This takes work and time.

What I can tell you is this: painful feelings associated with trauma and tragedy will not lessen or go away if you do not deal with them. In fact, it is my experience that they only become repressed and the unconscious feelings stemming from the System 1 regions of our minds become more intense. This results in overwhelming feelings of numbness, sadness, depression, and anger, which can lead to sleeplessness, changes in eating patterns, workaholism, excessive drinking/smoking/drug use, and physical ailments such as headaches and stomach problems.

Know that all of these are normal human reactions to traumatic situations. We are not robots who lack emotions. However, there comes a point when our quality of life, our relationships, and our future are affected to such a negative degree that we cannot see a way out. This is when we need to exert our freedom to choose. We can either stay stuck in the circumstances of our tragedy or make a conscious decision to shift our thinking to System 2 and create a new life.

Retell Your Story

Acceptance is the final stage of grief. At this stage, an individual is ready to move to the next phase of their life. They have come to terms with what has happened and understand that life will never be the same. They also are ready to create a new and meaningful narrative for their future.

I began this chapter with my good friend who has a child with a severe genetic abnormality. While upon discovering the heartbreaking news she felt alone, betrayed, and frightened, that is not where her story ended. Metaphorically speaking, eventually she acclimated to her new environment, learned a new language, and found this strange, new city more beautiful than her wildest expectations. One remarkable aspect of her reframing process was her involvement in a nonprofit advocacy organization that fights for the rights of the disabled. This woman's new narrative empowered her *Self* and her family with a new perspective filled with joy, love, and meaning.

When memories and expectations wired into our brains as superhighways are challenged by traumatic situations, we have to surrender those visions for new ones. And we have to stop traveling on those same superhighways that are stuck in the past. In chapter 4, I discussed how critical your *Self*-directed thoughts are in the rewiring process. This is especially true as it concerns reframing a tragedy. The thoughts you create around a new and positive vision of your life are powerful. When you repeatedly act upon them, you begin to rewire your mind. You destroy the superhighways that carry the old narrative and build new ones that transport you to a new story. And you create a new life, perhaps even a better one.

I love what psychotherapist Nira Kfir wrote:

> Crisis means a change in the flow of life. The river flows relentlessly to the sea. When it reaches a point where it is blocked by rocks and debris, it struggles to find ways to continue its path. Would the alternative be to flow backwards? That is what a person in crisis craves, to go back in time. But life doesn't provide a reverse gear, and the struggle must go forward, like the river, with occasional pauses to tread water and check out where we are heading.[5]

Josh's Story

My twenty-nine-year-old son, Josh, has experienced great adversity in his young life. Just hours before he was to play in the semifinal game of the North Carolina state high school football play-offs as a senior, my young daughter and I were watching a movie in the local theater. We had trouble concentrating as our minds reeled with anticipation of the upcoming game. During the film, my phone buzzed from different numbers, some I didn't recognize. Finally, after the tenth missed call, I called one of the numbers. Whoever was on the other line told me my son had been in a car accident and was in the hospital's critical care unit, fighting to survive. Life would never be the same for the Chilton family.

The past twelve years have been quite a roller-coaster journey for all of us as we have struggled to understand and adapt to the barren destination where our airplane landed. Josh has courageously volunteered to tell his story in the following pages to offer hope to many of you so that you can begin to move forward in your own journey.

Even in writing this chapter, I am keenly aware that our family is still in the process of reframing this tragedy. But as you already know, the point of rewiring our minds is not about perfection; it is about making progress. Here is Josh's story in his own words.

On the day after Thanksgiving in 2003, I was driving in a downpour to see my girlfriend when I lost control of my Honda Accord and hydroplaned into a tree line. This particular day was supposed to be one of the highlights of my life up to this point. The anticipation was tremendous as I was to play middle linebacker for my high school football team, the Mount Tabor Spartans, in the semifinals of the state play-offs against the West Charlotte Lions.

The fear I felt in the moment before impact still haunts me today. The crash happened so fast that I didn't even have time to brace for the impact. What took place after the crash is hard to explain, and I likely will never understand it on this side of heaven. All I remember is feeling like I entered into a timeless state, a peaceful place that I had never experienced, even in my dreams. It was similar to testimonies of near-death experiences that I had heard or read about. In some surreal way, it felt as though my life was being evaluated. I can't articulate this moment in words, but it was certainly a gateway between two worlds, the living and the non-living, as well as a portal between two distinctly different lives for me. I entered as the football star who was popular in school with a beautiful girlfriend and a bright future filled with goals and aspirations and exited into a frightening and unfamiliar world where death lurked and pain was all that made sense to me.

When I regained consciousness, someone was talking to me, but I had no idea what was going on. I was in shock. I began to piece together that I had been in an accident. I was in my car feeling the cold rain run down my face and a pool of red blood splash in the raindrops. I was terrified and struggled to breathe. I tried to move, but I couldn't get up. It was then that I realized I couldn't feel or move anything below my waist. I fought to stay conscious, as it felt like I was fading away. It was in this condition that I remember the rush of adrenaline throughout my body as it called on every reserve I had to survive. I asked the person if I was okay, and he told me not to move, that help was on the way.

I do not recall being removed from the car, but I do remember being in the ambulance. My phone, somehow still in my pocket, rang repeatedly. I knew it was my girlfriend and eventually convinced the EMS attendant to answer and tell her to meet us at the hospital. I'll never forget the pain I felt as the shock wore off. I couldn't stop screaming and begged the doctors to put an end to all this pain. Once I was stabilized, they took me to surgery. The rest is a blur.

My teammates and coaches won the game 28–3 that night, not knowing if I would live through the evening. I still have the game ball signed by everyone in a glass case at my house. Over the next few days, the ICU was flooded with hundreds of visitors. I dozed in and out of consciousness from surgery and medication, but the faces of certain family and friends stuck out. The outpouring of love and support from family, friends, and strangers was overwhelming. Doctors told me my spine was crushed and that the oxygen had been cut off to my nerve cells in my spinal cord, causing them to die. I was paralyzed from my waist down and would likely remain that way for the rest of my life.

I insisted on attending the state championship game two weeks later. I wanted to show the entire community how thankful I was for their love and support. I was transported to the stadium via ambulance and lay on a stretcher with an ICU doctor and nurse by my side. It was only after watching my teammates take the field that I began to process what had happened to me. They could play and I could not move. A reporter from a local television station interviewed me during halftime. I made a bold proclamation in spite of my diagnosis. I told the reporter that one day I was going to walk again.

Since the accident, I've struggled to find and establish a new identity. The first stage of grief is denial. Denial was the greatest obstacle to my recovery. I wanted my old life back. As a result, I rebelled against my situation and refused to take care of this new body that I hated so much. As my denial deepened, I became angry, depressed, and self-destructive. I alternated between completely isolating myself and abusing drugs and alcohol. I also struggled with deep-rooted emotional and chemical addictions.

For years, I was bitter and resentful. I was mad at God for causing my injury. At that point in time, I thought the day of the accident was the day God took from me the life I deserved. I was mad at my girlfriend for not sticking by my side. I was mad at my friends and other people for living normal lives, playing ball and making plans for the future. I was obsessed with the whys and the what-ifs. And I often contemplated suicide but was too afraid to go through with it. As long as I continued to not accept my circumstance, I could not even begin to think of redesigning a new life.

Many times I even demanded a miracle from God. As time slipped away, absent of that miracle, hope and faith dwindled. My addiction to alcohol and drugs grew deeper by the day. I bitterly watched my prior life pass me by through the lens of social media. My friends graduated college and moved on to start families and careers. Many reached out to me, but I didn't reach back. I was ashamed because I could not deliver on my promise to walk again.

My dad has described System 1 in overdrive throughout this book. Tragedies such as mine place people in an ultimate form of System 1 in complete overdrive. Because of my deep resentment for the way my life had turned out, I could do anything to numb my pain. I compromised my morals and values with little regard for consequence. I put myself in dangerous situations in an attempt to feel anything other than what was coming out of my mind.

On December 3, 2014, my destruction finally caught up with me. I had only a hundred dollars to my name. I had pawned all of my electronics. I had borrowed all the money that I could from my parents. So I did what made the most sense. I used every last dollar to buy my last gram of drugs. After snorting it, I waited to die.

I was coming down from the high when my mother knocked on my door. She would occasionally stop by my house to check on me to make sure I was still alive. I had constantly tried to convince my family that the root of my problems was depression and not addiction. They had no idea how deep I was into this underworld of drugs. When she found me by myself in a dark room, malnourished and shaking from fear of the unknown, she began to cry and said that I needed to get help. I stared at the ceiling weighing her words and my options.

For the first time in my life, I could not think my way out of my situation. It was time to surrender. I finally told my mother the truth—that I was addicted to drugs and I wanted help. I will never forget the feeling of relief that came over me when I finally admitted the truth to my family and myself. Don't get me wrong, I was scared and dreaded the withdrawal process at rehab, but my desperate determination and desire for change were strong.

To me, reframing tragedy meant changing the way I looked at my accident. In order to move forward, I needed to rewire my brain to create a new story for my life. I needed to believe I could be a new person. I had to be honest with myself and my situation. I needed to surrender my previous expectations of what my life would be. Letting go of our false sense of control and surrendering our will is difficult, but it is the only way we can be free. I am now beginning to see my accident not as the day I lost it all, but as the day I was allowed to live.

I am still searching for complete acceptance with my injury. There are times when my mind tells me that all is hopeless and I should give up or self-destruct. I struggle with this fight every day as I try to change the way I think and continue to work hard at figuring out my new life. However, I am confident that my new approach to life will produce progress in my development as a happy and productive person.

Like most of us, I'm a work in progress. And while I don't have all the answers and am in the thick of change, I do know that I desire a full life, one in which I do not fear being an active participant. Transformation is happening, though slowly. As we say in the program, one day at a time.

I do not know your story, where you have been, or what you are going through. But if you are in the dark shadows of hopelessness, as Josh was, my deepest desire is that his story will encourage you to believe that no matter your situation, there is hope. Miracles typically do not take the form we expect or ask for. But they are nevertheless out there waiting for us. The God I believe in is a God who provides second chances for our brokenness. No matter the source of or kind of tragedy we experience, he gives us the capacity to reframe our tragedy so we can have new, magnificent lives. It is like the apostle Paul wrote: "And we know that in all things God works for the good of those who love him" (Rom. 8:28). Our heavenly Father desperately wants to give us life again.

Reflection: The Pathway to Rewire Your Mind

1. Name a particularly traumatic life event that you have been through. What was your initial reaction? How did that emotion or behavior morph over time?
2. Have you struggled with the loss of a dream or unmet expectations of life? Have you come to terms with what your life looks like right now? Why or why not?

3. How important is faith in your life? Has it helped you cope with the emotional aftermath of a painful or tragic situation? If not, do you see any possible ways that faith can be a source of strength?

4. What have you learned about your *Self* after experiencing a loss or devastating situation?

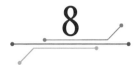

8

Facing the Greatest
Challenge—Parenting

I think when a man finds good or bad in his children he is seeing only what he planted in them
after they cleared the womb.

John Steinbeck, *East of Eden*

Laura, a single mother of three kids, divorced her abusive
husband four years ago. Since the separation, her sixteen-
year-old son, Brian, has continued to abuse Laura in the
same pattern he observed in his father. Brian is particularly
good at manipulating and controlling Laura by using to his
advantage her guilt and low *Self*-esteem issues arising from
the failed marriage and broken family.

For example, it is common during dinnertime for Brian to
mouth off to his mother for no reason. When Laura verbally

reprimands him, he initiates an explosive fight that ends in his saying something like, "You're just a dumb witch who can't do anything right. It's no wonder Dad had an affair." Brian's outrageous behavior inevitably leads to Laura grounding her son. In a predictable abuse cycle, over the next couple of days, Brian apologizes to his mother multiple times, attributing his atrocious ways to the stress of the divorce and transition into a new school. Then he tells her over and over how much he loves her. Brian's seeming remorse is always draped in dramatic fashion worthy of an Academy Award. Expectedly, Laura experiences tremendous guilt and removes or lessens his original punishment. A few weeks later, the cycle repeats.

When Laura and Brian meet with Brian's counselor, Laura feels even more guilt. The therapist emphasizes the profound stress Brian is under and says it is understandable and even normal that the boy would lash out in such abusive ways. Brian uses the counselor's sympathies to continue his destructive behavior and push Laura's guilt button at home.

I believe the main reason this woman remains stuck in this abusive pattern is because her System 1 is stuck in overdrive, a response to the abuse she suffered in her marriage and her guilt associated with the breakup.

As I will discuss below, women are initially the primary caretakers and protectors of their children, sustaining them in the womb and beyond. Though System 1 primitive survival instincts to protect, nurture, and sustain are powerful and positive traits, they often spin out of control as a child transitions into adolescence. These instincts together with difficult external circumstances cause overactive fear, guilt, and shame responses that can cripple parents and prevent them from raising a child in a healthy and positive way.

In the following pages, you will learn the difference between toxic parenting fueled by a hyperactive System 1 and a healthy upbringing activated by System 2. This is not a how-to parenting crash course. My aim is to inspire you to recognize the areas you may need to work on through counseling or other means in order to lead your children well.

Unconditional Love

I believe the underpinning of most parental struggles is the confusion over unconditional love and conditional acceptance and the roles they play in the parent-child relationship. Erich Fromm, in his classic book *The Art of Loving*, offers much insight about the unconditional love a parent has for a child.

Before I continue, I want to acknowledge that in modern society, due to the high number of divorces and fragmented homes, both mothers and fathers often are forced to take on multiple roles in their child's development. However, before we explore these dynamics, I want to provide a child developmental road map with two parents in traditional roles from the perspective of Fromm. This then will help us better understand the dual roles we must often play in other situations.

Before a child is born, he is biologically attached to his mother for sustenance. After birth, the attachment bond continues on both an emotional and a physical level. A baby is helpless and vulnerable to the world around him, dependent on his mother for nutrition, warmth, and security. For all intents and purposes, mother and child are still one.

As the child grows and develops, his view of the world around him expands. He begins to understand that he is a separate entity apart from his mother and that people, objects, and places exist outside of his immediate line of sight. In time, the child begins to learn how to handle his environment to make things more pleasurable and less harsh. The mother remains at the epicenter of this learning experience. She continues to feed the child when he is hungry, respond when he is crying, and nurture him with her maternal instincts. Perhaps most importantly, the child begins to understand he is loved. These powerful and natural feelings and activities arise from our System 1 survival instincts to protect our young. Collectively, they are very important for the healthy development of a child and if not carried out properly can lead to numerous System 1 dysfunctions (such as attachment issues, discussed in the next chapter) as the child becomes an adult.

A mother's love is natural and beautiful, unadulterated and whole. It cannot be acquired or manufactured; it just is. Fromm writes of the growing bond between a mother and her young, "All of these experiences become crystallized and integrated in the experience: I am loved. I am loved because I am mother's child. I am loved because I am helpless. I am loved because I am beautiful, admirable. I am loved because mother needs me. To put it into a more general formula: I am loved for what I am, or perhaps more accurately, I am loved because I am."[1]

This is what is known as unconditional love. A child does nothing to deserve love; he simply has to be. He does not need to reciprocate his mother's love but only respond to the love that is offered. Receiving unconditional love creates in him a solid sense of confidence, security, and well-being.

While a good father is able to provide unconditional love to his child, up to this point, his experience is different from a mother's. His role as dictated by biology is less connected to the child. He provides support and nurture, but because he was never physically attached to the child or able to provide sustenance through his body, in the first few years of development, the child has not yet depended on him for survival. But the father is not completely useless, of course. His System 1 instincts do facilitate initial bonding with the child, but his primary focus is on providing for and protecting the family unit.

As the child grows and becomes more independent, beginning to walk, talk, and learn how to fit into his world, the father has the opportunity to play a more vital role. Fromm offers that in an ideal situation, the father "represents the other pole of human existence; the world of thought, of man-made things, of law and order, of discipline, of travel and adventure. Father is the one who teaches the child, who shows him the road into the world."[2]

Unconditional love is one of the deepest needs of the human spirit. Children desperately need to feel they are loved simply for being who they are, not for what they do. When this does not happen, their subconscious System 1 tells them they are not loved and are simply being used. This produces great insecurity in children that is carried over into adulthood.

My friend Joyce grew up in a strict Eastern European household. Her mother would hug and tell her "I love you" only on rare occasions, typically on holidays and birthdays. The only time Joyce's mother doled out compliments or nurturing behavior, however slight, was when Joyce won high marks at violin competitions, washed the dishes without being told, or others remarked, in her mother's presence, on how thin or pretty Joyce looked. When the opposite was true, Joyce's mother reverted to her cold, distant self. This aloof and conditional display of love caused Joyce to believe for years that she was worthy of love only if she performed well, looked good, or did the right things all of the time.

Clearly, unconditional love is important to a child. With it, a child has a head start on life. Such a child is more confident, is better equipped to form healthy relationships with others, and has a generally positive outlook on life.

Conditional Acceptance

Though parental unconditional love tells a child he is and will always be loved, this does not mean a parent accepts a child's rebellious, destructive, defiant, or harmful behavior. There is a vast distinction between unconditional love and conditional acceptance. It is critical that parents understand this difference and how to merge the two if they are to raise a child who can reach his potential as an adult. From a parental rewiring perspective, the System 1 instinct to provide for and protect a child must be subjugated to the parent's System 2 understanding of the importance of boundaries, discipline, and responsibility.

As a child approaches adolescence, his brain and body mature. He interacts with the world in meaningful ways. He goes to school. He makes friends. He develops interests. He is exposed to external influences such as societal pressures, different cultures, contrasting worldviews, entertainment, education, and media. It is critical that a child be provided with guidelines, rules, and a moral foundation in order for him to pave a meaningful way in life in the midst of these outside forces.

Conditional acceptance shows a child how to treat others in a fair and respectable manner and that this is expected of him. It teaches moral principles and standards he must abide by. This love is patient and tolerant but at the same time persistent and uncompromising. It exacts consequences for unacceptable behavior and is unwavering in discipline. If you have made clear to your teenage daughter to stay away from drugs, enacting a no-tolerance policy, and find a bag of marijuana in her room, conditional acceptance will follow through with the forewarned punishment. You can reinforce that your love is steadfast in spite of this behavior, but you must also enforce appropriate consequences. Otherwise, your daughter will never learn right from wrong and general responsibility.

I know many parents who, for different reasons, tolerate their child's disobedience, lack of respect, or misdeeds. Some turn a blind eye. Others refuse to exact discipline for fear the child will do worse things. Whatever the reason, these parents act upon unconsciously exaggerated System 1 feelings that tell them their child is perfect or come up with what they believe is a reasonable answer for why their child is misbehaving.

The foundation of conditional acceptance is the capacity to honestly appraise a child's behavior. Bring to mind the slippery slope of excuses I talked about in chapter 6. Excuses are detrimental to a child's overall development and particularly their moral development. It is destructive to respond to bad behavior by saying things like:

"Oh, it's not her fault."

"He didn't mean to do it."

"Her friend so-and-so is much worse."

"He was just having a bad day."

These excuses not only blind a parent but also hurt children in the long run. Not being held accountable and responsible for their actions prevents children from becoming independent, responsible, and capable of living morally meaningful lives. Children who are parented in this way cannot develop into autonomous people. They may be intelligent but lack qualities such as discipline, determination, courage, and strength that are necessary to successfully navigate life. As they become adults, many become helpless, dependent on others to do things for them or make them feel a certain way. They constantly need to receive from others without giving back of themselves. Worse still, many develop narcissistic personalities and become completely focused on themselves with little to no capacity to express empathy for others.

Merging Two Loves as a Child Develops

Although it is critical to impose initial limits and consequences early in a child's life, Fromm says the transition from unconditional love to conditional acceptance should take place when a child is between six and eleven years of age. This progression is highly dependent on our capacity to engage System 2 executive control because it feels natural to protect our children by excusing or denying their behavior. As discussed above, biology dictates that the mother and child have the strongest connection in early childhood. Fromm posits that in an ideal situation, transitioning to conditional acceptance is when a father should take on a much more prominent role in parenting.

This is not to say that before this time the father has been absent or disengaged from his child's development and must now step forward to help the child understand boundaries and accountability. In fact, this is the time when both parents must shift their child rearing philosophy from mainly provision and protection to a conditional acceptance model. Together, they are responsible for helping the child understand that there are real and definable expectations and responsibilities in and outside the home. The child needs to understand that while he will always be loved, defiance and rebellion will not be tolerated.

I acknowledge we live in a world in which families are in crisis. The structures and expectations for family life have changed dramatically over the past one hundred years. With single parenthood[3] and stepcouples[4] on the rise, it is now common for a child to be raised under those household dynamics. While the undercurrents of family structure are constantly changing, I also recognize that unhealthy parents are everywhere, even within intact marriages. Whether you are a single parent, have a spouse who is rarely home or is disconnected in the relationship, or are happily married, it is both necessary and possible to forge a healthy fusion of unconditional love and conditional acceptance for your child.

I will speak from my experience of being a single father for eight years. As my children grew up, I adopted the "5 to 1 rule" from researcher John Gottman in his bestselling book *Seven Principles to Making Marriage Work*. Gottman posits that couples in successful and lasting marriages have more positive interactions than negative ones, a ratio of roughly five to one. In other words, there are five times more positive actions (praise, gratitude, physical affection, compliments) than negative ones (judgment, criticism, accusations). I believe this principle works just as well in parent-child relationships.

I tried my best to balance the difficult conversations with my children (setting strict boundaries, discipline, punishment) with more positive interactions (expressions of love, nurturing, affirmation, and even play). I didn't keep a running scorecard in my head, but this principle of balance was always at the forefront of my parenting goals.

So while I instilled in my children discipline and responsibility, and rarely let them get away with not being accountable for their actions, I was intentional about building positive experiences. I played with them. I made up bedtime stories about fictional characters. I read to them. Almost every night, we played a round of the basketball game HORSE complete with smack talk. I often told them how much I loved them and was proud of them. While these practices got more difficult as they turned into teenagers, I believe my love early on provided a foundation that made discipline and boundaries down the road much more effective.

Modern Parents on System 1 Overdrive

Now that I have addressed a balanced approach to loving and raising a child in a healthy way, I want to focus on three areas of modern parenting where I see that System 1 is in overdrive. Parents who do not set strong boundaries and discipline guidelines fail their children. That is the real tragedy—not that their kid didn't get accepted into a certain class or school. I was in a "retarded" building for two years, for goodness' sake!

While parenting styles are unique to the individual—and I certainly am not criticizing specific methods—I believe there are general System 1 responses in overdrive that are damaging this generation of young people. I have met far too many kids who appear to have narcissistic, entitled, and abusive mentalities and behaviors that often lead to addiction and failure to thrive. We don't intentionally raise our children to be this way. It happens when parents will not execute System 2 control over their emotional dysfunctions for the sake of their children.

Parenting by Guilt

Think back to the opening of this chapter, where I introduced Laura, the single mother paralyzed by guilt. This woman represents a large number of parents, particularly women. Guilt is typically produced by the System 1 fear of not being a good enough parent. This fear, in addition to rationalization, is a major enemy to raising healthy, productive, capable, and independent children in our modern society.

We feel guilty for getting divorced. We feel guilty for staying married. We feel guilty for working long hours or not working enough. We feel guilty for buying our kids too much or too little. We feel guilty for not giving them the right hand sanitizer, for not enrolling them in certain schools, for not providing them with a nuclear family unit. We feel guilty for being too strict, for letting them (or not) have sleepovers, for living in a certain zip code. This list is endless.

Whether our fear of not being a good enough mom or dad comes from our own insecurity or from external influences such as the neighborhood parents, so-called experts, or the latest child studies, guilt remains a powerful System 1 emotion. Whatever the source, it prevents parents from making the decisions necessary to raise mature and independent children.

Some guilt is normal for parents. Most moms and dads every now and then have a certain amount of regret or wish they would have done things differently. We are humans, after all, and make mistakes. But when this emotion is in overdrive, it is all consuming. We end up doing things that are ultimately detrimental to our children's well-being. We buy them too much stuff and influence them to become materialistic. We minimize boundaries and, consequently, do not instill in them personal responsibility. We give in to their demands and create narcissistic and entitled children.

Guilt may be a parent's most selfish System 1 emotion. In order for parents to feel better, they make incredible compromises as to what's best for their children. While they may feel temporary relief from guilt, what they are really doing is stunting their children's emotional development. And in the long run, these actions will have devastating effects on their children as well as on the child-parent relationship.

Overparenting

Also known as "helicopter parenting," being excessively involved in every aspect of your children's lives in order to protect or guarantee their success is a parent phenomenon that was initially recognized on college campuses in the early part of this century. Parents had hovered over their children to such an elevated degree that first-year students were terrified to launch into the college experience without their parents beside them every step of the way. These kids were accustomed to Mom or Dad making sure life was easy for them so

166

that they never experienced failure or hardship. These parents always came to their kids' rescue at the slightest evidence of a challenge. They problem-solved difficulties for their children. And many of them overextended themselves in the process. In turn, this type of parenting produced young people who lacked independence and leadership skills and were spoiled and lazy. While this type of parenting may have been given its name on college campuses, it shows up much earlier than those young adult years.

A helicopter parent is the hotheaded parent at Little League who always gets hostile with the umpire because he feels the guy made a bad call and now his son is out of the game. It is the parent who spends weeks helping her child fill out college applications and write essays and then tells her friends that "we" are going to Columbia. It is the parent who does his son's science project for him so he will take home the first place ribbon. It is the parent who ensures her kid has the perfect teacher, the perfect coach, the perfect friends, the perfect combination for a perfect life free of stress and adversity of any kind. Overparenting tells children they don't have to work that hard on their own because Mom or Dad will make sure that in the end they win.

If you are a parent of a young child involved in sports, you probably have witnessed the equivalent of every player on a team getting a trophy regardless of how hard they practiced or how good they are. Coaches do this so no one gets their feelings hurt. Everyone comes out a winner! This reminds me of a story told by the Greek historian Herodotus. A man asks a tyrant how to efficiently govern his city. The tyrant demonstrates his advice by going through his fields, cutting down the tallest ears of wheat, and throwing them away.

This destroys the best part of the crop. It seems crazy, but the tyrant is conveying his advice that the best way to control a city is to execute everyone with outstanding gifts, especially gifts for leadership. Rewarding every child in sports equally, regardless of performance, has this same effect of cutting down the outstanding children and discouraging hard work and excellence.

If we give everyone the same praise or the same reward no matter how hard they work or practice, then work and practice become meaningless. While uniform attention is designed to show everyone that they are equally special, it does a great disservice to children later in life when they study at a university and are placed in a 150-student chemistry class taught by a professor who doesn't know or care who they are. At that point, these young adults will feel alone and not so special. Worst of all, they will not have developed the coping skills to handle this difficult situation.

I recently read Jean Twenge's and Keith Campbell's book *The Narcissism Epidemic: Living in the Age of Entitlement*. I was blown away by the empirical evidence pointing out the damage we are doing to our children via overparenting. The book emphasizes recent studies that clearly show alarming increases in narcissistic personality traits among young people. Twenge states, "Narcissism increased just as fast as obesity over the past 25 years, and a study today shows that it is twice that rate since 2002."[5]

In a 2014 UCLA study of college freshmen nationwide, only 45 percent believed it is important to "develop a meaningful philosophy of life." Forty-three years earlier, the percentage stood at a high 73 percent. That same year, only 37 percent of college students prioritized the goal of making money; by 2014 it was 82 percent. Young people seem to care less about purpose and meaning and more about being financially well-off.[6]

The science is in. Hovering over our children and relieving them of autonomy and responsibility will hinder them from having a life of purpose and joy. It is not our job to make life easier for our kids. In fact, it is quite the opposite. It is our job to challenge them and equip them with the tools they need to adapt and succeed.

Years ago, I gave an academic talk before a prestigious group of scientists at Johns Hopkins University. During the Q & A at the end, a very famous scientist asked me a strange question. "Dr. Chilton, I know you hail from a rural region of North Carolina. What motivated you to go from there to one of the top levels of academia here at Hopkins?"

I didn't even have to think about the answer. "My parents," I replied. "I had a strong mother who loved me enough to insist that I work hard both in the tobacco fields we farmed and in school. During summers and on weekends, Dad got me up at 5:00 a.m. to work in the fields. Even when the temperature soared to nearly 100 degrees, as it often does in August in North Carolina, we continued to work. And while my parents supported me emotionally, it was up to me to fight my own battles—and there were many—particularly in school. With that kind of upbringing, getting to Hopkins was the easy part."

Parental Division

Conflict between parents on how to raise their children can cause incredible tension. This divide can stem from contrasting parenting styles, childhood upbringings, personal beliefs, and parenting goals. A mother may be more lax in her approach to discipline versus her husband, who rules with an iron fist. A husband may feel undermined in his role as protector and life teacher by a wife who insists on controlling every aspect of their children's development. In cases of divorce, each parent may enforce different rules, depending on who has custody that week, which leaves children confused. In cases of blended families, household guidelines may not be clear and guilt for placing children in a new situation is at a premium.

Clashing parenting goals can destroy a couple's relationship and offer the opportunity for a child to manipulate the situation to the detriment of all. However, because a child only understands his current System 1 needs, both parents, whether married or divorced, must be adults, shift into System 2 reasoning, and do what is right for the child and the family as a whole.

I am not naïve. I do understand there is no easy fix. But if this is something you struggle with, I highly recommend you see a licensed therapist to find resolution. This is imperative. Your child's future is at stake.

It's Not How You Start but How You Finish!

Raising good kids is a long and arduous process. You should never judge your effectiveness as a parent too early in their upbringing. I think about my four adult kids who, growing up, were very much like their father, a wild rebel at heart. Out of respect for their privacy, I won't detail all of the challenges we went through, but I am proud of each one and the meaningful lives they have developed over the years.

I admit that when my kids were between roughly fifteen and twenty-one years of age, I couldn't make sense of their actions or realities. As a scientist who spends his days providing structure to the mysteries of the universe, I was troubled that I couldn't understand my children fully. It seemed some days they loved me, others days they hated me. Some days they were happy, other days they were upset. Some days they were motivated, other days they were lazy. Some days they were angels, other days they were, well, you get the point. The constant flux of emotions and drama was not easy to manage or even figure out.

However, this is a great example of how my understanding of brain plasticity turned out to be a huge advantage. My frustration at their behavior shifted when I began to consider that the human brain does not reach full maturity until the mid-twenties. Knowing that the developing brain of a child and teenager undergoes considerable wiring and rewiring in a very short period of time and then prunes the very same nerve connections only to start again helped me view their unpredictable emotions and actions in a different light. It helped me make sense of their erratic behavior. As they progressed into their twenties, I knew that much of their brain activity was moving from back and mid (System 1) regions to front (System 2) regions so things were going to get better and much more logical. And I also understood that my steadfast unconditional love / conditional acceptance approach to their actions was playing a critical role in how their brains were being wired as adults.

Even under the best of circumstances, teenagers will have difficulty understanding expectations and risks, managing emotions, and handling relationships. The biology and psychology of raising kids is a messy business, and we must view it as such or we will drive ourselves crazy wondering what we are doing wrong and how we could do better.

At this point in my life, I have four adult children and an eight-year-old grandchild. Needless to say, I have been around the parenting block. If you are a parent of young children, I encourage you not to ride the roller coaster of your kids' emotions and actions because their brains and emotions are changing and developing so rapidly that they don't know who they are at any given moment. If you fuse your emotions with theirs, you will live in a world of constant chaos and anxiety. Trust me, it is much easier to be a caring and objective coach from the sidelines than a coparticipant in a teenager's craziness.

A few months ago, I was at a Christian writers' conference. I happened to be discussing this chapter with a few of the participants. A wonderful couple pulled me aside and quietly, with a hint of embarrassment, said, "We are incredibly concerned about our sixteen-year-old son. He just revealed to us that he is an atheist. What should we do?"

I told them that at one time or another all four of my kids decided they were atheists. Today, however, they have embraced the spiritual life and live rooted in God's love. I gently put my arms around this couple and said, "Congratulations! Your son's a thinker. He's decided that his faith is important enough for him to think about. You know, when C. S. Lewis was fifteen, he decided he was an atheist. And look at what happened to him. Relax, God's got this."

My point is that as children learn, grow, develop, and begin to think for themselves, which is critical in order for them to navigate effectively in life, you shouldn't stay fixed in freak-out mode. If your System 2 *Self* can reduce your exaggerated System 1 fears and instincts associated with child raising, you will be able to give your children the best possible gifts during this tumultuous time: emotional stability and joy. While definitely challenging most of the time, parenting can actually be a great deal of fun. Parenting in a balanced manner creates more laughter and less tension. This in turn provides children with the assurance that while they may be confused and occasionally mess up and have to pay a price for it, in the end, everything will be okay. And, more importantly, they will still be loved.

Reflection: The Pathway to Rewire Your Mind

1. Name three values you hope to hand down to your child. How are you accomplishing this?

2. Growing up, what was the most sacred lesson your parents taught you? Have you passed this down to your own child?

3. What are some areas you need to work on when it comes to unconditional love or conditional acceptance?

4. Honestly assess your current parenting style. Now compare your parental strategies to the character you see being formed in your child. What are some positives? What are some of the challenge areas that can be revisited?

9

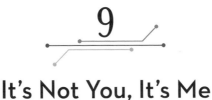

It's Not You, It's Me

Truth is everybody is going to hurt you: you just
gotta find the ones worth suffering for.

attributed to Bob Marley

Relationships are messy. We all know this to be true. While
reality TV is an accurate though disturbing looking glass
into unhealthy relationships, we don't need this famous clan,
that big-city housewife, or a very public divorce of a famous
athlete to tell us relationships today are an outright mess.

According to Jennifer Baker of the Forest Institute of
Professional Psychology in Springfield, Missouri, almost 50
percent of first marriages, 67 percent of second marriages,
and 74 percent of third marriages end in divorce.[1] We are
destroying each other one marriage at a time. But marriage
isn't the only crucible in which relationships are tested, tried,

and ultimately strengthened or ripped apart. Our parents can drive us crazy. Some of us can't stand our co-workers. Others have serious sibling rivalry issues or trouble getting along with in-laws.

I contend a majority of this discord is due to the System 1 fears, anxieties, and expectations we bring into a relationship. Relationships, with their multitude of survival responses, are fertile battlegrounds as the System 1 feelings and reactions from each individual involved differ and collide.

When we enter into relationships of any kind, whether intimate, friendly, or familial, we bring with us an array of both instinctive and default System 1 responses that stem from previous relationships and past experiences. At first glance, it seems a miracle that any relationship lasts. And to a large degree, it is impossible for any to flourish when both parties are overwhelmed by System 1 in overdrive.

The Differential Difference

In chapter 5, you learned that at our core we humans are lonely and long to be in a relationship. As Erich Fromm puts it:

> This desire for interpersonal fusion is the most powerful striving of man. It is the most fundamental passion; it is the force, which keeps the human race together, the clan, the family, and society. The failure to achieve it means insanity or destruction—self-destruction or destruction of others. Without love, humanity could not exist for a day.[2]

How differentiated an individual is will play a critical role in their capacity to have healthy relationships. In chapter 2, I introduced the concept of differentiation and the health issues that arise when cells do not mature properly. Differentiation at an individual human level also refers to maturation, especially with regard to the balance of System 1 and System 2. For instance, if you struggle with intense loneliness, anxiety, or obsessive thoughts, you are likely to maintain even an unhealthy or toxic relationship to avoid being by yourself. The more indispensable you view a relationship, the more you will go to great lengths to tolerate and preserve it.

Undifferentiated people are driven by System 1 fears, worries, feelings of isolation, and *Self*-doubt. Like undifferentiated cancer cells in the human body, undifferentiated people have characteristics that render them potentially harmful to themselves and others. They are often needy, selfish, and insecure. In many cases, they have major trust issues and very controlling personalities. Forming relationships with such people is likely to create a high level of drama and overall toxicity.

However, before you start accusing your significant other, your parents, your best friend, or your sister of being undifferentiated and poisoning the well of relationships, it is best to recognize that, like the past, you can't change others. Rewiring starts when you shift your focus to explore *your own* level of differentiation.

How well do you use System 2 reasoning over your System 1 feelings and behaviors? Have you compromised your values, social life, or family life to work sixty hours a week just to feel successful or make more money than you need? Do you feel you must exert control over everything and everyone, especially your family and friends, or else things will just not work out? Does your excessive care for others (including your children) impede their development, compromise your healthy boundaries, or cause you to say yes when you should say no? If you said yes to any of these questions, you just might have a System 1 issue.

Remember, it's not about others; it's about us. If you have trouble finding and maintaining healthy relationships, it is time to *Self*-reflect. As clinical psychologist Lisa Firestone says, "The most valuable aspect of recognizing a lack of differentiation is that once we're aware of it, we can start to question cynical or hostile attitudes toward ourselves or toward others. We can recognize these attacks from someone else's point of view and develop a deeper understanding of ourselves by identifying where these thoughts come from."[3]

Markers of Differentiation

I believe there are at least three primary components that determine an individual's level of differentiation in the context of relationships. These include how well one:

1. knows and expresses a true *Self*,
2. understands and manages System 1 emotional dysfunctions,
3. loves.

Consider again the highway illustration used in chapter 4. You will notice that when System 1 and System 2 are in balance, these three primary components are the off-ramps from System 1 to System 2. They are fundamental to pruning back System 1 and beefing up System 2.

At the end of this chapter, I offer you an opportunity to rate your *Self* in these three areas to ascertain your overall level of differentiation, but for now let's explore what these markers mean.

Know and Express Your True Self

A key to maintaining healthy and meaningful relationships is being able to remain your *Self*, a distinct, separate individual with unique strengths, as you connect with another. You do not change who you are to please the other. You communicate your thoughts, feelings, and opinions in a positive and nonhostile manner. You do not rely on approval from another to make simple decisions like what to wear or the right thing to say. You are free to share your opinions, ideas, and beliefs. You engage in hobbies that tap into your interests and passions, not just activities a friend, co-worker, or lover prefers. You acknowledge and celebrate your unique talents and strengths, what sets you apart. You maintain a healthy independence.

In a relationship in which both parties are differentiated, each individual brings a unique identity and personality, passions, talents, strengths, and values to form a powerful and distinct entity that is much stronger than either of the individuals alone. This cannot occur if the two are in a constant battle for control of the relationship. Toxic friction will move the union in an unhealthy direction rather than add meaning and purpose.

When healthy independence does not exist, two people fuse together to become a weaker, less effective union and can develop the trappings of codependence, a common emotional dysfunction in relationships. Preventing this merger is one of the most difficult challenges of connecting with another. In differentiated relationships, however, each *Self* encourages and nurtures the other.

Understand and Manage System 1 Emotional Dysfunctions

The second differentiation component necessary for healthy relationships is how well an individual understands and manages their System 1 emotional dysfunctions formed from negative or unhealthy past experiences. There are two in particular that plague and destroy a large proportion of relationships: transference and attachment.

Let's begin with transference. Sigmund Freud, the founder of psychoanalysis, was the first to describe how all people unconsciously transfer feelings from past relationships onto new relationships. Modern psychologists define transference as "a tendency in which representational aspects of important and formative relationships . . . can be both consciously experienced and/or unconsciously ascribed to other relationships."[4] This comes from primitive System 1, which is designed to protect us from potential threats and can explain why we continue to repeat certain relationship patterns.

For instance, a woman with a dominating father or ex-husband may believe all men are the same; in her mind, they are all controlling and even abusive. In doing so, she may unconsciously respond to minor conflicts in her current relationship with familiar behaviors and feelings (instigating defensive arguments, being afraid). The frequency and intensity of her responses may ultimately sabotage what could have been a beautiful relationship. Likewise, a man who was betrayed by his best friend as a teenager may view new acquaintances and even old friends with deep suspicion and mistrust. Transference is harmful because due to the magnified negative thoughts, fears, and behaviors, an individual cannot be their true *Self*.

The key mechanism underlying transference is that the characteristics of the most important people in our past are stored in our System 1 memories in multiple regions of the brain. Unconsciously, we relive the most relevant (painful or pleasurable) aspects of our early relationships. They covertly color much of our lives and particularly our interactions with others. Because memories are unconsciously triggered, we tend to automatically relate to people based on our past experiences. We assume others will have similar traits, even though they have no association or link to our past.

Think about a time you met someone new and thought something about that person reminded you of a significant individual from your past. Did you think or say something like, "He reminds me of my uncle" or "She is just like my best friend from college"? Now think how premature your assumption very well could have been. In fact, it was likely nowhere near the truth.

Transference sets up a *Self*-fulfilling prophecy in which everyone fits into a past pattern that naturally becomes the mold for the future. In this way, we unknowingly create past-derived outcomes in the present and the future. In reviewing my own life, I believe that transference has been my single most destructive System 1 tendency in relationships.

Attachment is defined as "a deep and enduring emotional bond that connects one person to another across time and space."[5] It is most often associated with our relationships with our parents. Parent-child attachment styles become so deeply internalized that we bring them into our most significant relationships, particularly our intimate ones. Statements such as "She has daddy issues" or "He's a mama's boy" ring true. If a man was spoiled rotten as a child by his mother, he may seek the same kind of behavior in women when looking for a mate. This is why a woman entering into a potential long-term relationship should be aware of the interactions her partner had as a child with his mother. Likewise, a man should understand the relationship between a woman and her father. In the book *Triumphs of Experience*, author and Harvard University psychiatrist George Vaillant summarized many of the most important outcomes of the longest study of adult development. Beginning in 1938, the Harvard Grant Study followed 268 male Harvard undergrads and their emotional and physical health, relationships, coping strategies, religions, political stances, and careers for over seven decades. The study interviewed not just the participants but also their families and friends.

With regard to childhood experiences, two characteristics predicted general outcomes during life and into old age, "cherished" and "loveless." Men in the cherished group had warm, positive childhoods and felt loved and accepted by their parents, particularly by their mothers. In contrast, the loveless men had distant parents and little nurturing, gentleness, and love from their mothers. Their childhoods lacked warmth and emotional support.[6]

The cherished men who had healthy interactions with their moms had huge relational advantages that lasted a lifetime. They were four times more likely to have lots of friends and loving and supportive social networks at age seventy.[7] On the other hand, the loveless men had great difficulty in relationships and an impaired capacity for intimacy. Compared to the cherished men, the loveless men smoked more and had higher incidences of substance abuse, were eight times more likely to have suffered depression, and made 50 percent less money.[8] These statistics reveal the tremendous impact of child-parent relationships.

That said, some men in the study who didn't have the best of childhoods were still able to experience success, joy, and meaning in relationships and in life. As a wise old country man once told me, "Ski, you can choose almost everything, but you can't choose your relatives. You are stuck with them." If your parents were neglectful, overindulgent, or abusive, you can recover from these issues. Seek counseling, join support groups, read helpful books, and do what you have to do to find and maintain relationships with supportive, nurturing people.

Love

The third trait of a differentiated individual in relationship is that they know how to love. According to Erich Fromm in *The Art of Loving*, there are at least five types of love: brotherly love, motherly love, *Self*-love, love of God, and erotic love.[9] Brotherly love is loving and caring for most others. Motherly love is the unconditional love of a mother for her child. *Self*-love is the capacity to love one's true *Self*. Love of God springs from our desire to be in union with our Creator and Sustainer. Erotic love is the craving to be in complete connection with another and is where two separate individuals become one.

It is critical to understand that these five loves are distinct, cannot be substituted one for another, and require different types of loving approaches. Though they may have overlapping characteristics, a love for a sibling is different from a love for one's *Self*. A love for God is different from a mother's love.

A particularly confusing issue in many marriages is the comparison of motherly love and erotic love. I recently had a friend tell me that after she gave birth to her first child, she knew she would never experience love like that again. She then added that the love she had for her child was so much stronger than her love for her husband. I disagreed. Measuring a love for a child compared to a love for a spouse is not useful or appropriate. Even though the term *love* can be ascribed to different relationships, there is a difference. In a family, you love your spouse and your children in very different ways, not one more than the other. Not recognizing this fact can have detrimental consequences for a marriage. This is one of the reasons why couples experience tremendous gridlock when they start a family. Understanding the different kinds of love helps differentiated individuals form and maintain healthy relationships.

I believe the biggest roadblock to loving well is understanding what true, sustainable love is, particularly in intimate relationships. Many believe it is a feeling that comes and goes. Others believe it means being *Self*-sacrificial to the point of losing one's identity. Another major misconception is viewing love as a state of being rather than a choice and a series of actions.

When two people start dating, typically it is the woman who at some point asks the man, "Do you love me?" or "Are you in love with me?" The question is usually met with initial silence, with the man looking like a deer caught in headlights. I am now beginning to understand why this question means so much to most women. My wonderful girlfriend has taught me that little girls view love as an idyllic state of being, a mystical world in which two perfect people reside in a state of permanent bliss. It is the fulfillment of the Cinderella story, being swept away by Prince Charming and living happily ever after "in love." I know from personal experience that what is going on in the minds of little boys or men is nowhere near the level of sophistication of this fairy-tale image, which is why men get tripped up by the question.

The unspoiled vision of love that many women—and, in their own ways, men—have gets shattered quickly when Prince Charming becomes Prince "why did you leave your underwear on the floor for the millionth time." I urge you to read 1 Corinthians 13:1–8 at least once a week as a reminder of the characteristics of true love:

> If I speak in the tongues of men or of angels, but do not have love, I am only a resounding gong or a clanging cymbal. If I have the gift of prophecy and can fathom all mysteries and all knowledge, and if I have a faith that can move mountains, but do not have love, I am nothing. If I give all I possess to the poor and give over my body to hardship that I may boast, but do not have love, I gain nothing.
>
> Love is patient, love is kind. It does not envy, it does not boast, it is not proud. It does not dishonor others, it is not self-seeking, it is not easily angered, it keeps no record of wrongs. Love does not delight in evil but rejoices with the truth. It always protects, always trusts, always hopes, always perseveres.
>
> Love never fails.

As I introduced in chapter 5, another obstacle to loving well is the belief that love should be reciprocated. How often have you thought that giving love, doing or sacrificing for another, means giving something up and expecting something in return?

> If I watch my neighbor's dog while she's on vacation, I'll have to take time out of my hectic schedule. She will owe me.

> I hope my mother really appreciates my taking her to the doctor again. I'm missing another lunch with my girlfriends. Maybe she'll cover gas this time.

> My husband wants me to have his department over again for the holiday party. Maybe I can get him to make it up to me by buying me that watch I really want.

When we view love in this manner, we consciously or unconsciously believe our giving will ultimately dry up the well. Our sacrifices, our doing, our loving will cause us to be spent. This model of love is not sustainable because we expect a return on our investment.

True love involves a very different economy. When we give without expectation of anything in return, God gives love in abundance back to us in different ways. As you know, I learned the paradoxical nature of *Self*-sustaining love by connecting with beautiful orphans in Africa. I admit, it is often much easier to love strangers, especially children, compared to the people we are closest to. This is because we know both the positive and the negative parts of our spouses, friends, and family members, and they know ours.

Still, love is always possible. When we engage System 2 and temper overactive System 1 impulses and reactions, we understand how to set and keep boundaries and remain our authentic *Selves* in any relationship. And we know how to love and give in a way that will leave our cup running over, not running on empty.

Finally, I must point out the difference between this love and codependency, which I touched on earlier in this chapter. When two people connect at whatever cost in a desperate attempt to eliminate loneliness, individuality is lost. Both parties play a role in this type of unhealthy relationship.

Codependence presents in a variety of ways: an overprotective and jealous boyfriend (dominator) who refuses to let his girlfriend (dominated) do anything or go anywhere without his permission; a mother (enabler) who constantly gives her drug-addicted daughter (enabled) money; a manager (taker) who doesn't respect his co-worker's (giver) boundaries and constantly gives him more work to do without adequate compensation. Whether the codependent relationship is between a parent and child, two friends, or a husband and wife, men and women equally participate in destructive activities, some more than others.

The need to control another is a System 1 primitive instinct that manifests itself as domination and manipulation of another person to maintain power over one's own environment and relationships. When this response is in overdrive, relationships suffer tremendously. In the worst case, a person who dominates a relationship exploits, hurts, and humiliates the other while remaining completely insensitive to the damage they cause.

Let's talk about the flip side of codependence. Individuals in a relationship who are the dominated, the enabler, or the giver instinctively respond to loneliness and fear of separateness by offering themselves in very unhealthy ways. Melody Beattie, author of *Codependent No More*, wrote, "Codependents are reactionaries. They overreact. They under-react. But rarely do they act. They react to the problems, pains, lives, and behaviors of others. They react to their own problems, pains, and behaviors."[10]

Differentiated individuals will approach a relationship with true love and kindness, not in a codependent manner. This means being sensitive to the others' needs, setting healthy boundaries, and cultivating the union with their strengths.

System 2 in Action

I believe we are to love everyone—and sometimes this means in a healthy way from a healthy distance. In practice, loving others can be extraordinarily difficult in certain situations.

Loving others does not mean we ever unconditionally accept the actions of others that are destructive, harmful, or unhealthy. Differentiated people use their capacity to understand others to determine potential threats of a relationship to their well-being. Their System 2 monitors, analyzes, and predicts an outcome by observing another's character, actions, behaviors, and responses. In an intimate relationship, this surveillance may take place in the midst of intense System 1 feelings of attraction, lust, romantic love, and the primal need to fill the void of loneliness. This makes it all the more difficult, but it is possible.

System 2 reasoning in differentiated individuals can beautifully balance all the System 1 emotions behind the cliché "Love is blind." People who can make sense of their own emotions and at the same time see the behavior of another for what it is will not be swayed by System 1 excuses ("But he can change"), wishful thinking ("Things will get better"), insecurities ("Maybe I need to try harder"), or fear of being alone.

I am amazed how wise people who love and want the best for us usually have the capacity to analyze our relationships much better than we do. I can't tell you how much easier my life would have been had I heeded my mother's advice on relational issues. Then again, I probably would not be writing this book and sharing with you my colorful stories.

In 1997, Oprah Winfrey and Pulitzer Prize–winning poet Maya Angelou were having a heart-to-heart about the famed talk show host's unhealthy relationship at the time. Oprah opened up about how she felt constantly let down by the man she was dating. Angelou responded, "Why are you blaming the other person? He showed you who he was. . . . Why must you be shown twenty-nine times before you can see who they really are? Why can't you get it the first time?"[11] The poet's words are earth-shattering for me. They stuck with Oprah, who, over the years, amended this wise advice to say, "When people show you who they are, believe them the first time."[12]

When your System 2 overrides System 1 attraction and loneliness, you will believe a man the first time he tells you he doesn't want a serious relationship. You will believe a woman the first time she treats you like she doesn't care.

A few years back, I had a provoking conversation with a female acquaintance. She told me that after her husband's third affair, she was so exasperated that she screamed at him,

"Who are you?" He looked at her with eyes cold as ice and for the first time told the truth. He answered, "I am who I've always been."

In other, nonintimate relationships, you will believe the family member, the colleague, or the friend when their actions speak louder than words. You will see the true colors of a sibling who always tries to borrow money without any intention of paying it back. You will see the true colors of a co-worker who constantly tries to pawn off work on you. You will see the true colors of a friend who is always too busy when you need a listening ear.

Our System 2 understands that we cannot change the past or another person's character. People change and rewire themselves only when they desperately want or need to. When others show you who they really are and their characteristics are not compatible with the kind of life and future you want to create for your *Self*, run! If you choose to stay and get pummeled by the destructive consequences, there is no one to blame but your *Self*.

When to Walk Away

I love reggae music and particularly Bob Marley, so I was destined to start one of my chapters with a quote most often attributed to this talented musician: "Truth is everybody is going to hurt you: you just gotta find the ones worth suffering for." It is as inevitable as the sun rising in the morning that due to humanity's imperfect nature, even the best of us will hurt and disappoint another. Whether in the context of marriage, friendship, or family, someone you love will cause you pain. The opposite, of course, is true as well.

This often involves silly but annoying things like being incessantly nagged by your partner for forgetting a chore. Pain goes deeper with more serious issues like reneging on a promise; belittling or disrespecting another; verbal, emotional, or physical abuse; adultery; or harmful addictions. In the most destructive situations, such as addiction or abuse, how does a differentiated individual judge whether or not to sever ties? How do you know who is "worth suffering for"?

In the case of intimate relationships, including marriage, one of the biggest expectations people have is that their partners will change. They will somehow stop hurting you and others, stop cheating, stop lying, stop drinking, and somehow clean up their act. Unfortunately, most times the cycles of behaviors only continue. As I have discussed throughout this book, System 1 fears, emotions, and behaviors are extraordinarily deep-rooted because they are wired to DNA and brain circuitry that is difficult to change. Unless a person hits bottom as a result of intense stress and pain or develops a deep desire to change, they can't and they won't.

Understand that I do not encourage divorce. I believe God gave us the gift of marriage, and he intends for spouses to love and support each other until the day they die. I also strongly believe he can miraculously save marriages in ways I cannot even begin to explain or even understand. However, if you are in a relationship that becomes particularly destructive, it is imperative for you to seek safety so that you can take care of healing your *Self*. Seek professional, expert, and spiritual counseling. It may be necessary to separate to allow for time to heal. You may have to get out of the way to begin to work on issues on your side of the road and provide your partner time and space to do the same.

I am not a licensed counselor, nor do I have all the answers. If you need it, I highly recommend you seek help for your relationship outside of this book. What I can tell you is that getting divorced or even separated does not entitle you to go out and find another partner only to allow the same System 1 issues to destroy another relationship. There is a reason that the divorce rate markedly increases with each subsequent marriage. As we will discuss in chapter 12, until we surrender our fears and insecurities to God and allow his power to change us, it will not be possible for us to find love and contentment outside of our *Selves* in *any* relationship, let alone marriage.

What about friendships? Or relationships with family members, including parents? What approach do you take if your best friend constantly makes unreasonable demands or does not respect your boundaries? Or if your mother or father constantly criticizes the way you dress, chides your parenting skills, or engages in negativity in every conversation you have? While it is easier to recognize unhealthy behaviors in a friendship and "break up" with a toxic friend, how can one be differentiated with a difficult family member?

I believe that relationship survival in close familial unions depends on making a choice of whether you can live with the other person's System 1 stuff without demanding or hoping they change. This is more difficult if you have children who are being directly affected by this unhealthy individual. For instance, if you have a parent who is verbally abusive and occasionally goes off on inappropriate tirades in front of your kids, the solution to set clear boundaries for the well-being of your children is obvious.

In less volatile familial relationships, differentiated individuals can observe the System 1 reactions of relatives without allowing themselves to become emotionally involved or manipulated. In this setting, we must understand that there is no chance for others to change unless they deeply desire to do so. Minds wired for extended periods of time have circuits that can by definition produce only one outcome. Once we understand that unhealthy individuals close to us have no free will and react in the only manner available to them, it becomes much easier to simply observe and not get involved in their activities.

Reflection: The Pathway to Rewire Your Mind

1. Have you ever maintained an ongoing relationship with someone even though it was unhealthy or toxic for the mere reason that you did not want to be alone? How did the relationship end? If you broke it off, what was your breaking point?

2. Do you have (or did you have) any codependency issues in any of your relationships (whether with friends, family members, or even your spouse)? How does (did) that element affect the relationship as a whole and you as a person?

3. Write down your most significant relationship at this time. List three roadblocks that prevent you from being differentiated in that relationship. How might you approach and ultimately remedy those challenges?

4. Take a look at the "Differentiation Index" below. Rate your *Self* in the three components of differentiation as it concerns relationships. Where do you stand? What is your overall score? What areas could use improvement?

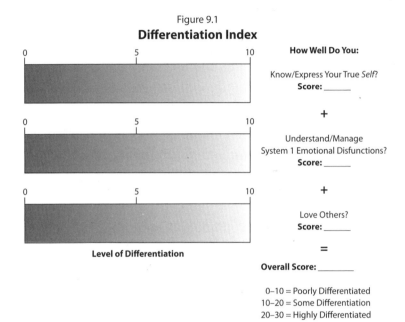

Figure 9.1
Differentiation Index

How Well Do You:

Know/Express Your True *Self*?
Score: _____

+

Understand/Manage
System 1 Emotional Disfunctions?
Score: _____

+

Love Others?
Score: _____

=

Overall Score: _____

0–10 = Poorly Differentiated
10–20 = Some Differentiation
20–30 = Highly Differentiated

Level of Differentiation

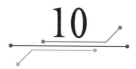

10

The Gift of Intimacy and Sex

> Human sexual desire is the most complex form
> of sexual motivation among all living things. It's
> a combination of genetic programming and vari-
> ables of life experience, producing the utmost
> sophisticated nuance and variety of sex on the
> face of the planet.
>
> David Schnarch, *The Passionate Marriage*

In the 2012 movie *Hope Springs*, Kay (Meryl Streep) and
Arnold (Tommy Lee Jones) have been married for thirty-one
years. They live a safe, monotonous, routine-driven life. Each
morning Kay dutifully cooks Arnold the same breakfast he's
had for the past three decades, one sunny-side-up egg and a
piece of bacon, while he reads the paper. After chowing down
his grub, Arnold leaves for work, and Kay does the same.
Day after day this marriage cycles around work, sleep, meals,

and watching the Golf Channel. Spontaneity, intimacy, passion, and sex do not exist in their world. Although Arnold loves his wife, he is clearly oblivious of this fact, hypnotized and quite content with his quiet though bland life. In contrast, Kay desperately desires change. Deep within, she is a passionate woman who longs for a marriage bursting with intimacy and steamy sex.

In one of the first scenes, Kay is disappointed when Arnold leaves for work without acknowledging their thirty-first wedding anniversary. She expresses this sentiment to a co-worker later that morning, asking if change in a marriage absent of intimacy, affection, and passion is even possible.

Her co-worker doesn't offer much hope. "Change your marriage? What do you mean? Like you mostly eat in on Fridays then you eat out, or you're at each other's throats then suddenly you're Cinderella and Prince Charming. . . . No, you marry who you marry, you are who you are. . . . Why would that change? . . . For that to happen it would have to be so bad that somebody was willing to risk everything just to shake things up, but then it might not come down your way. . . . Nah, marriages don't change."[1]

Determined to create a better marriage, Kay ignores these cynical words. She dips into her savings account and books a week of intensive marriage counseling with a renowned therapist, Dr. Bernie Feld (Steve Carell), in the sleepy New England town of Great Hope Springs.

After a very difficult and often hostile first session, Dr. Feld says to the couple, "You two have come here to try to restore intimacy to your marriage . . . to find ways to communicate your needs to one another . . . to cultivate intimacy and to develop the tools to sustain that intimacy going forward. The first step in rebuilding a marriage is tearing away some of the scar tissue that has built up over the years. . . . It can be very painful, but it's worth it. I like to think of . . . the metaphor of when you have a deviated septum, and you can't breathe . . . you have to break the nose in order to fix it."

I love this movie and believe every couple, especially ones that are experiencing difficulty, should watch it. It is inspiring to watch Kay, who for years has played the role of a shrinking violet, reach the point where she is no longer willing to live the rest of her life sacrificing intimacy and sex for the sake of a comfortable and safe marriage.

What Is Possible

I believe sex and intimacy within a committed, covenant, and monogamous relationship are two of God's greatest gifts to humanity. We all know what sex is, the physical offering of ourselves to one another. Intimacy is a bit more complex. It is being emotionally close to your partner, being able to completely share your inner world, who you really are, with that person. It is about being vulnerable and connecting honestly and in-depth in all areas of your life. Intimacy can include sensual expression; sharing thoughts, feelings, and ideas; and being aware of who you and your partner are as individuals. It is possible to have sex without intimacy, but a central premise of this chapter is that sex without intimacy is problematic. When two people are united in a committed relationship, they create a deeply passionate and transformational encounter that has the capacity to bring about closeness and differentiation in a relationship like no other human experience.

At their best, sex and intimacy blend the best parts of System 1 and System 2 emotions and behaviors in a mystical manner that powerfully transitions our intimate relationships from mundane to extraordinary. When System 1 instincts such as sexual desire, spontaneity, creativity, and longing for connection dynamically merge with System 2 qualities such as imagination, fantasy, and diversity, two differentiated individuals have the powerful capacity to transcend space and time and move much closer to a realm of great spirituality.

Evidence for this type of intimacy exists in the Bible, particularly in the book Song of Solomon. A baptism by erotic fire, the text drips with intimate sentiment right from the opening line:

> Let him kiss me with the kisses of his mouth—
> for your love is more delightful than wine. (1:2)

Other lines include:

> I belong to my beloved,
> and his desire is for me.
> Come, my beloved, let us go to the countryside,
> let us spend the night in the villages. (7:10–11)

These incredibly beautiful, sensual, and provocative verses articulate the passionate level of communion God had in mind when he designed committed relationships.

In addition to our capacity to connect with God, this type of intimacy with another person is what makes us truly unique and human. In profoundly spiritual acts of bonding, your commitment to your partner is conveyed through actions, not just words. You enter a capsule of sexual space, and time stops. Here you and your partner can experience deep connection and transformational joy and love. You come alive by every heightened sensation, not just in your body but also in your mind. The climax of orgasm is almost secondary because the connection is so profound. And with increasing intimacy over time, this communion grows stronger, even outside the bedroom, as you begin to relate to each other in new ways. You experience exciting, new adventures while laughing and playing together like carefree children running through a beautiful meadow.

Some of you may be frustrated at this point, rolling your eyes and saying, "Okay, okay, Dr. Ski. This world of mountaintop or romantic-novel-type sex may be the goal, but my marriage looks nothing like what you are describing. I'm stuck on the ground floor with Kay and Arnold."

I hear you! And I want to encourage you that however lifeless or passionless your sex life may be right now, it can be rekindled. You can experience powerful and transformative intimacy and sexual desire. Bear in mind, there is no formulaic, one-size-fits-all plan or ten-step road map to achieve this pinnacle of connection. The differentiation process looks different for every couple.

I also acknowledge that married couples endure different seasons and medical conditions in which sexual intimacy and function change. I do not expect any couple to be swinging off chandeliers a week after a wife gives birth or if a spouse is injured or has fallen sick.

If you have a physically, mentally, or emotionally abusive partner, I encourage you to seek safety and counseling immediately. Trying to forge a healthy and passionate sex life in the midst of a relationship that has serious and even life-threatening dynamics is simply not possible nor recommended. Get help from a trusted counselor, professional spiritual advisor, mentor, or support group. Also, if you or your partner suffers from a medical condition that impedes sexual function, consult with a physician to guide you accordingly.

Lastly, know that it is impossible to fully address something as complex as sex and intimacy in a few thousand words. I am honored if reading this book starts you on a journey and you and your spouse have a desire to move beyond the scope of this book. My favorite author on this topic is world-renowned sex and marriage therapist David Schnarch. I highly recommend his books *The Passionate Marriage* and *Intimacy and Desire* to continue the push forward.

The Ebb and Flow of Love

Several recent studies focus on the brain chemistry and brain regions involved in sexual desire and intimacy. According to biological anthropologist and author Helen Fisher, when we first begin a romantic relationship, our brains buzz with activity. At this point, our attraction is more than a feeling. We experience a powerful set of System 1 instinctive drives. Fisher writes, "Like the craving for food and water and the maternal instinct, it is a physiological need, a profound urge, an instinct to court and win a particular mating partner."[2]

This initial stage of what we call "falling in love" is the biological process in action when we read a love story, watch a romantic comedy, or listen to a love song. It is the form of "love" that most of us automatically equate to true, lasting love. And that is what causes a world of problems in long-term relationships and marriages when the pink mist rises and we see each other for who we truly are, the good and the bad.

According to Fisher, falling in love typically involves three basic System 1 drives. It often begins with lust, the craving and yearning for sexual gratification, and then progresses to romance, a strong drive for the new partner. Finally, as the relationship progresses, attachment develops, the union between two people in a long-term, monogamous relationship that includes having and raising children.[3] Many scientists liken the one- to two-year stage of romantic love to temporary insanity. Biological studies show that during this time our cognitive function—the capacity to feel negative emotions, clearly assess situations, and evaluate trustworthiness—is markedly reduced as our brains are bathed in a euphoric cocktail of neurochemicals and hormones, including dopamine, vasopressin, and oxytocin.

Most of us question whether the System 1 emotions and behaviors of initial romantic love can be sustained. The fact is, biology dictates that they will likely (though not in every case) fade over time. Your heart may not continue to skip a beat when he calls. She may not always look her best every time you see her. He may stop bringing home flowers and whisking you off to romantic hideaways.

In the beginning of relationships, persuasive System 1 instincts centered on lust, attraction, and reproduction simply push us to find, pursue, and capture a mate and then conceive a child together. Breeding is vital to support the transfer of our genes from generation to generation. Alone, the System 1 desire to breed has little to do with and in fact can limit our capacity to have intimate, monogamous, and long-term relationships.

As people move through the falling in love stage, they begin to know their partners very well—the good, the bad, and the ugly parts, including morning breath, unbecoming bodily functions, annoying habits, irritating personality traits, and the like. They also learn the sexual habits and limits of their partners. According to Schnarch, sex between two people consists of the "leftovers" they each bring to the relationship.[4] The leftovers are the repertoire of acceptable sexual practices that each partner has decided they are willing to do according to their own sexual development. These leftovers can potentially create a barrier to sexual variety within a relationship. The full spectrum of knowledge they have about each other births familiarity, which can demystify or change one's initial lustful attraction and romantic love as well as create sexual stagnation and boredom.

Lust and romance will ebb and flow in a relationship, as change is the only guarantee in life. Undifferentiated individuals expect romantic love, sex, and passion to last forever without effort. They are disappointed when these things wane. For these people, the solution is obvious: end the relationship and find a new partner to fall in love with. Sadly, this short-lived cycle is doomed to repeat. An individual who does not understand this and is not committed to defining and differentiating their *Self* will possess a misguided and destructive hope that someday they will find the "right person" who will be interesting and sexy enough to sustain romantic love forever. Sadly, this individual will continue to be disappointed.

As I emphasized in the previous chapter, love is not a state of being or merely a strong feeling but a series of determined decisions and actions. Maintaining intimacy to continue on a journey of sexual development past the initial stage of romantic love and leftovers takes courage and work. When we exchange vows and say yes to a marriage of forever, part of that commitment includes saying yes to developing and growing in every facet of life, including intimacy and sexual desire. If you want to have powerful intimacy and sex with your partner, you must discard your Hollywood movie views and expectations of romance and love and develop a new model centered on a more differentiated *Self*.

Major Myths

Before I offer key components of developing your *Self* and your relationship so you can experience a heightened level of sex and intimacy, I must address three misconceptions that serve as roadblocks for many.

Sex is natural, and, consequently, great sex should come without much effort. It just happens, right? Wrong! Sexual desire is extraordinarily complex, especially as couples move from dating to a long-term relationship. According to biological anthropologist Agustín Fuentes:

> Every human brings with her or him a suite of embodied experiences to every sexual encounter and even to every thought, consideration, or fantasy about sexual encounters. At a minimal level this includes one's gender, the current gender expectations of his/her society and all the subdivisions in that society s/he belongs to, personal life history and past experiences and exposure to sexual activity, sexual orientation, and age, health, body image, religion, politics, economics, computer access, etc.[5]

I would add to these experiences the key differentiation factors discussed in the last chapter (how well we know and express our true *Selves*; our understanding and managing of System 1 emotional dysfunctions arising from our past; and how we love). Great sex, especially in a long-term relationship, is far from easy. In fact, it may be easier to coordinate all the systems on the space shuttle. I would quickly add, however, it is worth it!

Women are less interested in sex than men. This is a common myth that is simply unsupported by data. Helen Fisher examined ninety-three societies and found that men and women had roughly equal sex drives in seventy-two of them.[6] In his book *Intimacy and Desire*, David Schnarch offers that if the sex is good, women are often more interested in it than men. He also points out that wives are typically more sexually knowledgeable than their husbands.[7]

If you are a woman and feel insecure about not having a strong sex drive, know it is likely in you. I believe God intended sexuality to be a natural and meaningful expression of your *Self*. Intentional and unintended System 1 religious, family, or cultural influences send mixed messages that can quash sexual desire in women only to create intimacy struggles in their relationships later in life. A female's libido may also be diminished because of past experiences. I recently had a conversation with a woman who, as a little girl, was exploring her body when her mother walked in on her. The mother spanked the child and told her what a "bad" girl she was and never to do that again or she would go to hell. Over the years, this little girl carried with her a hard-pressed guilt surrounding sex that as an adult negatively affected her marriage. If you are struggling with any of these issues, know that God created you with a sex drive. This is nothing to be embarrassed or ashamed about. It's normal. It's healthy. It's a God-given gift. And it's a beautiful thing!

Sex is reserved for the young. I can't tell you the number of depressing articles I have read that told me my sexual prime as a male peaked at the age of eighteen. If this is true, then for me at the ripe age of fifty-eight, the party's been long over.

This fallacy was birthed from studies carried out and published in the late 1950s and perpetuated by women's magazines ever since. The original data establishing sexual peaks was determined by sexual hormone level measurements.[8] In men, testosterone levels topped out around the age of eighteen, and women's estrogen levels reached their apex when women hit their mid to late twenties. These hormonal mileposts have been called "genital prime" because they occur when our genitals respond most urgently to arousal. Don't let this discourage you. Genital prime has little to do with sexual prime. It is well documented that the greatest, most enjoyable, and most effective sex organ is the human mind.

Don't believe me? Look at some of the statistics. More than 50 percent of older adults say sex gets better with age.[9] Men between the ages of fifty and sixty-nine are the most confident with themselves and their capacity to perform sexually.[10] An article on sexuality in older adults in the prestigious *New England Journal of Medicine* showed that 54 percent of sexually active persons (ages seventy-five to eighty-five) reported having sex at least two to three times per month; 23 percent reported having sex once a week or more.[11]

These statistics astound me. Taken together, they reveal that your golden years, sexually speaking, may very well be ahead of you.

It's about You, Your *Self*

I believe there is a significant driver behind better sex as we age that is different from genital prime. The key is developing a differentiated, accepting, and confident *Self*. Like me, Schnarch believes the underpinning of passionate intimacy and sexual desire is the development, or the differentiation, of the *Self*. We must face our System 1 fears, attachments, control issues, complex histories of past sexual experiences, and romantic love expectations. Forging a passionate, intimate relationship begins when we take responsibility for our sexual and intimacy development.

Throughout this book, I have spoken about the importance of recognizing and confronting System 1 emotional dysfunctions as a result of childhood and later attachments, abuse, neglect, and other painful experiences. Our capacity to have intimate relationships depends in large part on the degree to which we have dealt with these issues. I have also emphasized that our capacity to love without expecting anything in return will play a key role in successful relationships. While these two key markers are essential, the most vital factor is the development of a strong, positive, and independent *Self* that taps into and builds on our strengths and does not rely on the acceptance of others, including a mate.

Schnarch says this type of *Self* is:

> Stable and flexible at the same time. . . . You can stretch it and bring out new facets, and prune old aspects that no longer fit you. You can change a solid sense of self when you want to, but retain your shape when others try to make you into who or what they want you to be. Flexibility and resilience

are the two basic and important characteristics of a solid sense of self.[12]

A differentiated *Self* is a confident *Self*. You are comfortable with who you are. You are free to share opinions and sexual desires with your partner. You have the courage to face the uneasiness that often accompanies sexual development. You are able to communicate with your partner without being defensive or judgmental. You are adaptable enough to make compromises. You are open. You are honest.

The journey toward experiencing a wild and passionate relationship with your partner is not about learning the hottest sex tricks or positions described in checkout line magazines. It is about the intimacy gained by two people learning to explore and discuss fundamental issues surrounding sex. It begins when you talk to your partner about intimate issues, struggles, or questions you have. It includes sharing hidden sexual desires or past experiences that may hinder you from letting loose in the bedroom. Since I will not be offering step-by-step advice or solutions for your particular issues, I encourage you to read the above-mentioned books *Passionate Marriage* and *Intimacy and Desire* for specific information.

I am well aware that openness of this magnitude may frighten some readers. You may be thinking, "What if my husband thinks I'm weird or a pervert?" "What if my wife rejects me or is turned off by what I have to say?" Maybe your fear has to do with cultural or religious expectations, a history of sexual abuse, being rejected by or losing a partner, or simply being paralyzed by the cycle of routine you have become familiar with for the past however many years. At this point in the book, I don't have to remind you that these are all System 1 feelings and thoughts that come with a predictable set of behaviors. In the past, they may have been important for your protection. Now, if you are in a covenant relationship with a partner of solid character who you trust will not physically or emotionally hurt you in any way, these System 1 fears serve no purpose and are roadblocks to pleasure.

That said, there is always risk in being vulnerable. The film *Shadowlands* chronicles the story of C. S. Lewis and his first and only love, Joy, a renowned poet. The couple married in 1956, when Lewis was fifty-eight years old. Sadly, a mere four years later, Joy died from bone cancer. In the movie, Lewis makes a profound statement: "Why love, if losing hurts so much? I have no answers anymore: only the life I have lived. Twice in that life I've been given the choice: as a boy and as a man. The boy chose safety, the man chooses suffering. The pain now is part of the happiness then. That's the deal."[13]

Love as well as sexual development cannot exist without vulnerability. Love cannot stand in its full power without the possibility of pain or rejection. While the absence of *Self*-expression and openness will guarantee a safe ride, it will likely be an unfulfilling and boring one. "That's the deal."

Codevelop with Your Partner

As you develop your *Self*, becoming more aware of and remedying your insecurities, hang-ups, and other issues with sex and intimacy, you are ready to codevelop with your partner. Sex between two differentiated *Selves* combines the carnal features of the primitive mind and reptilian brain regions with the loving, inspirational, and imaginative facets of the neocortex. Sex produces experiences that powerfully re-wire our minds, replenish our spirits, and reinvigorate our relationships. Sex in this manner is loving, adoring, hot, erotic, and even carnal all at the same time. This *will* keep boredom at bay.

I acknowledge that readers of this book will be in different phases of life and sexual development. Like Arnold in *Hope Springs*, your spouse may have no interest or not be ready to take this journey with you. Or maybe your spouse needs to first work on personal struggles or challenges to be ready for the adventure.

For those of you who are committed to a willing fellow adventurer who desires to climb up this mountain with you, it is critical to establish a new equilibrium. Form an alliance with your significant other. Commit to embarking on the exciting adventure of sexual development together. Notice I did not say each individual in the relationship fuses with the other in codependency; rather, each participates in the differentiation of the other's *Self*.

Begin stoking the fires of intimacy by gaining a better understanding of who your partner is (their hopes, dreams, fears, wants). Take some time to talk with each other without children and not about paying bills, taking out the garbage, or little Johnny's soccer schedule. Either during a single conversation or over a period of talks, steer the conversation toward issues of sex and intimacy (desires, fantasies, what hinders you). It is important to do this without judging the other. Hold hands during this process to initiate an environment of love and safety. Once each person has felt the security of the other's embrace, sexual desire will begin to naturally arise.

Couples can move bit by bit through a whole spectrum of sexual activities ranging from simply touching to tender lovemaking to hot erotic sex and back again. Remember to take this journey one step at a time. If you are a year or even more into a sexual dry spell in your marriage, give your *Self* grace. You are not expected to light fires under your sheets this afternoon. This will take time and patience.

It is important to emphasize that because you both bring System 1 baggage to the process, you *will* reach impasses. You may be in the mood to share a fantasy and feel rejected when your partner is not excited to hear about it. Or you may have certain expectations of exploring a new sexual desire, but the activity falls short when it actually happens. Maybe in the process of explaining your feelings or wants you say something that comes off as condescending or even unintentionally hurts your spouse. Oftentimes, moving past sexual boredom requires the creation of sexual novelty. Someone has to initiate the conversation, which takes great courage. The new proposal may not receive instant validation and be outside the other's comfort zone because by definition it sits outside the "leftovers" category.

Whether conflict arises when you are simply being vulnerable and telling your partner your desire to reignite your sexual life or when you are expressing your sexual fantasies, it is normal and to be expected. This is when you must maintain a strong alliance. Both of you must be aware that intimacy and sexual development are critical and necessary if you want to turn back from boring sexual leftovers and redeposit passion and excitement into your marriage.

When gridlock occurs, maintain a stable and flexible *Self*. Don't let setbacks discourage you. Respectfully work through the issue together, whether on your own as a couple or guided by resources such as a counselor, books, or a workshop. It is important to keep the momentum alive, as the inability to move through conflicts surrounding intimacy and sex can be a major cause of divorce and affairs.

One of the most important tools to develop is the capacity to stay calm and *Self*-soothe your own hurts and desires instead of lashing out at your partner. Stay cool, don't overreact, and at the same time don't punish your partner by running away or creating distance that damages the relationship.

Keep in mind that when conflict is handled with grace, without anger, and wisely, it can strengthen relationships and rewire our minds more rapidly than other activity. Handling stress well induces genetic changes that alter how our brain genes are expressed, and this in turn alters brain wiring that beautifully coordinates System 1 and System 2 thoughts, feelings, habits, sensations, behaviors, and emotions.

Rewiring your mind in the areas of intimacy and sex will likely be the hardest, most frightening, and at the same time most exciting journey you will share with another in life. How you and your partner navigate the journey as the relationship and needs change has great ramifications for your life. Mishandle the journey, let a horrible childhood past rule your emotions, or take part in it dishonestly and in a manner designed to control or manipulate, and you may live a life without intimacy and sexual passion and miss out on many of God's greatest gifts to a marriage.

From the perspective of this chapter, know who you are, be true to your *Self*, and at the same time allow your *Self* to be vulnerable and flexible. Through this process, you and your partner can find love, connection, intimacy, and sexual desire in unimaginable ways.

Reflection: The Pathway to Rewire Your Mind

1. Are you emotionally present during sex? If not, what stops this from happening?
2. Can you be vulnerable with your partner and express your sexual desires? If this is difficult, why?
3. Do you and your partner experience conflict when it comes to issues of intimacy and sex? What do you see as your biggest obstacle to experiencing more passion?
4. How would you like to see your intimacy and sexual life improve? What are some steps you can take on your own and with your partner to make that happen?

PART 3

REWIRE

This section is about recovery. You will find intense and transformative *Self*-directed and *Self*-exploratory exercises designed to rewire your mind so you can find true and lasting change well beyond your reading of this book. Please understand that these three chapters offer a preliminary road map for the journey. While they focus on emotional rock bottom, surrender, and forgiveness, this is just a start. As mentioned in part 2, seek outside help in your areas of struggle.

One final thing: because of the intensity of the exercises offered in these final chapters, you will not find reflection questions as in previous chapters.

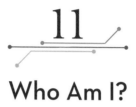

Who Am I?

> You are a slave, Neo. Like everyone else, you were born into bondage, born inside a prison that you cannot smell, taste, or touch. A prison for your mind. . . . This is your last chance. After this, there is no turning back. You take the blue pill and the story ends. You wake in your bed and believe whatever you want to believe. You take the red pill and you stay in Wonderland and I show you how deep the rabbit hole goes. Remember—all I am offering is the truth, nothing more.
>
> Morpheus, *The Matrix*

One of my favorite movies is the 1999 science fiction thriller *The Matrix*. I am fascinated by the scene in which Morpheus, the inspirational leader and teacher of the last of the truly free human race, offers his protégé, Neo, a choice between a red pill and a blue pill. With the blue pill, Neo will live with the rest of humanity in ignorance of a reality manufactured and controlled by the Matrix, a virtual computer-generated world run by machines. With the red pill, he can live in the "real world, " a life based in truth and filled with many unknowns and little control.

By now you are aware that you live in a matrix, not one generated by computers but highly influenced by your unconscious System 1 mind. Through the *Self*-discovery exercises offered in this and the remaining two chapters, I, like Morpheus, offer you a choice in how you want to live your life: stuck or free. I hope this book has convinced you that your only path to truth, love, and freedom is the "red pill." Only then can you discover your true *Self* and see how deep the rabbit hole goes.

The Bible contains eighteen verses that focus on walking in darkness. My favorite is Isaiah 42:16: "I will lead the blind in a way that they do not know, in paths that they have not known I will guide them. I will turn the darkness before them into light, the rough places into level ground. These are the things I do, and I do not forsake them" (ESV). This verse and particularly the word *darkness* make divine sense in light of the dominance of our System 1 unconscious minds.

God, through the words of the ancient prophet Isaiah, makes clear that we do not have to live imprisoned by System 1 emotional dysfunctions. Should we choose, he can turn the darkness before and within us into light. He can give us the power and the clarity to understand and express our true *Selves*. We can stop living as robots that react in predictable and destructive ways. We can lead the lives we desire.

Self-Discovery

In her book *The Top Five Regrets of the Dying*, Bronnie Ware beautifully documents the primary regrets and disappointments of hospice patients who have spent the remaining few weeks of their lives at home. When asked what they would have done differently, almost all said they wished they had had the courage to live true to themselves, not what others expected of them.[1] Sadly, when these patients reflected back on their lives, they realized how much time they had wasted doing neither what they loved nor what was most meaningful.

I can't help but wonder whether you can relate. Even in the absence of death's quickly approaching footsteps, can you honestly say you are living true to your *Self*—who you are at your core, weaving your strengths and passions into the tapestry of a meaningful life?

For me, three critical questions arise from reading about the regrets of the dying:

1. Is impending death the only event serious enough to prompt us to reflect on our lives to discover our true *Selves*?
2. How do we even begin to discover our true *Selves*?
3. Once discovered, how do we find the courage to express our *Selves*?

Let me first answer the initial question. You do not have to wait until you are given a death sentence to begin to discover who you are. You can start right now. The exercises in this chapter are a road map to help you begin the *Self*-discovery journey. With regard to the third question, the next two chapters, which unearth the bedrocks of surrender, forgiveness, and freedom, will encourage and strengthen you to express your true *Self*.

This process of *Self*-discovery requires honesty and depth, the activation of System 2 to ponder and excavate tough questions. Part of this means connecting with God through sincere, contemplative prayer. This "is nothing else than a close sharing between friends; it means taking time frequently to be alone with Him [God] who we know loves us."[2] If you are to truly know your *Self*, including the reasons behind your actions and feelings and the deeper meaning of your life, I believe you need insight from God. Who else knows you best?

If I asked, "Who are you?" how would you answer? I have found the default answer almost always centers on career or parenthood. "I'm an accountant." "I'm a mother." "I'm an actress." "I'm a doctor." "I'm a writer." This may be true, but even if you have the most important job in the world, like caring for your children, this is not who you are. Take it from a father who dearly loves his four adult children. If you define your identity by your children, once they leave the nest, you will be lost. Who we are is more than what we do. It is about what drives us, what motivates us, what fuels us to wake up each day with joy, meaning, and purpose.

In *Strangers to Ourselves*, Timothy Wilson says, "Many of people's chronic dispositions, traits, and temperaments are part of the adaptive unconscious, to which they have no direct access. Consequently, people are forced to construct theories about their own personalities from other sources, such as what they learn from their parents, their culture, and yes, ideas about who they prefer to be."[3]

In other words, your perception of your *Self* is largely based on a narrative you create from all the clues around (culture, family, social circles) and inside (unconscious feelings and behaviors) you. You may be so highly influenced by peer expectations that you shape a narrative that fits into what others perceive as cool or unique. However, there is a major rub in doing this. When the story you tell about your *Self* is not authentic and not consistent with who you really are, you get stuck between two conflicting worlds, your own *Self*-generated matrix. So the trick is to find the *real* narrative, the one deep within you that represents who you really are, how you really feel, and what truly brings meaning to your life.

The Incredible Power of *Self*-Narratives

The hidden, true *Self* within you desperately wants to be revealed and understood so you can put your life in context. The pathway to begin to make sense of your life and discover who you are is to tell your story. For nearly twenty years, James Pennebaker, esteemed professor of psychology at the University of Texas at Austin and author of several books, including *Writing to Heal*, studied the impact of writing *Self*-narratives on the mental and physical health of individuals. He discovered how the simple act of writing about our lives, including our honest thoughts and challenging experiences, is a pathway to healing, *Self*-development, and overall well-being.

Thousands of people representing all walks of life, from college students to maximum-security prisoners to new mothers, participated in these studies. These people wrote about the most significant events in their lives, their passions, and their deepest thoughts and feelings. This helped them create an understandable framework from which to view themselves, perhaps for the first time in their lives. Many became aware of the destructive roles their emotions and behaviors played in their most painful experiences. Others began to understand that their actions did not always accurately represent who they really were or who they wanted to be. Perhaps most importantly, these participants began to piece together when and why System 1 emotional dysfunctions started and how these toxic patterns over time quashed what they most desired for their lives.

I did this very assignment about ten years ago at the recommendation of a therapist. At first, I balked. It seemed like psychological nonsense, a waste of my precious time. Eventually, however, I surrendered and began to write. At first, the process was akin to Forest Gump going for a run that ended up lasting three years. I wrote for weeks. The narrative began with my deeply rooted feelings about being in the "retarded" building, the childhood bullying incidences, and the painful experiences of sexual abuse. The words poured out onto the page almost uncontrollably. This activity helped release my repressed feelings that desperately needed to be expressed so I could begin to be freed of their power.

On the flip side, I was surprised how difficult it was to write about what made me happy and gave me pleasure and joy. Oh sure, I could write about my "great" accomplishments and awards, the births of my four children, and other important events in my life, but these seemed nothing more than a list of positive memories. They told me little about my *Self*. Eventually, I discovered a common thread of helping those less fortunate than me. Yet while I had an inkling that doing that was a source of joy, purpose, and meaning, I wasn't totally sure.

Writing my story stirred within me intense emotions. On the one hand, I felt delight celebrating my life up to that point. On the other hand, I was overcome with deep sorrow at the hurt I had experienced and caused in others. But through these emotions, writing my story provided great insight about me as a person. I learned what I wanted most in this world and why I often felt a disconnect between my deepest desires and my behaviors. I believe the single greatest outcome of this exercise was that it exposed my depression and lack of joy despite my incredible efforts to be a good husband, a good father, a good scientist, a good Christian, and ultimately a good man.

This was a defining moment in my life. I began to realize how my past experiences made me feel inferior, unworthy, and unlovable and why during certain periods in my life I had acted so out of character in a desperate attempt to prove my value to my *Self* and others. Writing my story helped me identify and name the primary issue that was preventing me from being the person I wanted to be.

Your Turn: Exercise 1A

This first *Self*-exploratory exercise forms the basis for the remaining exercises in this chapter and the rest of this book. In a journal or on a computer, write down the story of your life. Focus on your most significant positive and negative events, experiences, and relationships.

Here are some questions to help you shape your thoughts. What experiences have brought you the most joy, pleasure, or meaning? What has caused you great pain? What are your greatest accomplishments and your biggest mistakes? Reflect on your most important relationships (with your parents, spouse, significant others, friends, relatives) and how they have affected your life positively and negatively. Also, consider your present and your future. What is going on now? Are you headed in a positive direction, or do you feel stuck? Is your life up to this point a reflection of the passions and goals you had when you were younger? What do you want to accomplish with the rest of your life? What do you believe is your biggest obstacle to making that happen?

Here are a few helpful tips as you get started.

- Find a time and a space that are safe and comfortable and you can write free of distraction. This might mean early in the morning, before your spouse or kids wake up, or late at night.

- Start with a time of contemplative prayer. Ask the Holy Spirit to reveal to you the truth of who you are. The Bible tells us, "'What no eye has seen, nor ear heard, nor the heart of man imagined, what God has prepared for those who love him'—these things God has revealed to us through the Spirit. For the Spirit searches everything, even the depths of God" (1 Cor. 2:9–10 ESV). What a testament to the power of soul-searching through the Holy Spirit.

- The only requirement or rule is that you are completely honest. This is important because the exercise is a tool to help you discover your *true Self.*

- There is no time limit to this exercise. You can write for fifteen to twenty minutes a day for a week or more or block out a bigger chunk of time and finish your narrative in a couple of days.

- Do not overthink this exercise or worry about punctuation or grammar. This is not an academic paper.
- If you get stuck, just write whatever comes to mind. Allow your mind to be free to express your *Self.*
- This may be an emotional experience for you. That is okay. As a matter of fact, it is good. Feel your emotions and write them down, however intense they may seem. If you feel you are starting to become overly emotional or depressed during this process, seek outside help with a counselor or professional spiritual advisor.

After you write your story, put it aside for a day or two and then reread it. Reflect on whether or not the narrative you created reflects the real you. *Self*-falsification serves no purpose and will only confuse you and prevent you from discovering who you are and moving in a direction that will improve your life. You can continue to write and revise this narrative if you choose.

You through Another Lens

I often get in trouble at work. I am a natural rebel, a fighter, passionate and outspoken, especially when it comes to causes I care deeply about. Others often perceive this characteristic as countercultural, politically incorrect, or even arrogant. Though I now appreciate this part of my *Self,* I did not always realize it. It came to a head several years ago when talking to a dear friend who studies human behavior. I was complaining to him about always being in the middle of controversy and the butt of much of my colleagues' criticism.

Exasperated, I said, "I hate arguments. I hate being in the middle of these scientific and health policy debates. And I hate having to take on all these issues. People hate me. I wish I could just be a normal faculty member, just like everyone else." I meant what I said. At least I thought I did.

My friend simply laughed and said, "Ski, I study human behavior every day, and I can tell you I've never seen anyone who enjoys taking on important causes more than you. You love being a rebel. You just don't enjoy the cost of being one."

He nailed me. If I wanted the story that I tell my *Self* about who I am to be more consistent, I needed to incorporate his view. He, like the people who know us inside out, saw as a character strength what I perceived as a negative *Self*-image narrative. Perhaps most importantly, he helped me realize I have a powerful unconscious response causing me to stand up for what I believe to be right. Today I embrace the nonconformist aspects of my *Self*. I consciously like the thought of leading rebellions with a purpose. This understanding helps me better withstand and even anticipate the criticism and pressure that go along with challenging the status quo.

Your Turn: Exercise 1B

As I just showed, the perceptions others have of us can be dramatically different from our own views. Many times they are even more positive! This is why it is important to get a second opinion on your narrative. It is quite possible that what you write down initially can be totally or somewhat off from who you really are. If this is the case, the exercise above is not going to be helpful.

Hence, your next assignment is to sit with a trusted friend, family member, counselor, or professional spiritual advisor and share your story with them. It is often helpful if this person knows at least part of your journey. It is also imperative that you feel safe sharing your deepest feelings and experiences with this person. Ask this person to read your story and give feedback. You can also verbally communicate your story if you don't feel comfortable providing the written narrative.

Ask this person how your narrative aligns with how they perceive you and your journey. Comparing how you view your *Self* with how those who know you do will often reveal positive and negative inconsistencies, including blind spots, hidden character strengths, and untapped passions. Add any new insights gained from this second opinion to your original narrative.

Take your time with this process. The accuracy of your narrative will be critical as you further explore your *Self* in the next two chapters.

The Passion Connection

As a professor in two large programs at Wake Forest School of Medicine, I interview dozens of PhD program applicants. My first question is always the same: "What are you passionate about?" While occasionally I will get responses like "becoming a great educator," "helping others," or "understanding the mysteries of science," I typically get a blank look. I find it fascinating that these students who have worked so hard to get to this point in their academic careers do not understand themselves well enough to know their passions and what will give their lives meaning. In chapter 5, I emphasized that for our lives to have meaning we must love others. Loving others may be as simple as checking in on a lonely older neighbor or educating a room full of high school students in mathematics. However, here is the catch: we do a better job of loving the world in our areas of passion. This is why it is important to figure out what they are.

Up until the past few years, whenever I was asked what I do for a living, I would say, "I'm a scientist" or "I'm a professor at a medical center." However, that response would typically move the conversation in a certain direction, and I would spend the next hour talking about whatever I was researching at the time. Now don't get me wrong. I love science and research. I have a natural penchant for these two fields that I have meticulously developed. However, I am not passionate about them for the sake of science and research. If they were not aligned with my real passion in life, they would bore me to death.

It took much of my life, including writing my *Self*-narrative and a very influential trip to Africa, to figure out what I am passionate about. During that time, I discovered that God has given me the gift of compassion. Consequently, I am passionate about spending my time on earth providing solutions to make people's lives better, easier, and more joyful.

My scientific knowledge and research are simply effective tools that allow me to carry out my passion and give my life deeper meaning. I spend hours in a laboratory not because I love being enclosed by four walls and surrounded by test tubes, sophisticated instrumentation, and high-power computers but because I am passionate about designing therapeutic foods for brain and immune system development for severely malnourished children in Africa and India. I have spent years researching brain plasticity not just to increase my knowledge base but to use this understanding to help others recognize what is not working in their lives and guide them toward a better way.

Most people can't answer questions like "Who are you?" or "What are you passionate about?" or "What gives your life meaning?" because often they are too busy and inconsistent with their *Self*-narratives to develop a meaningful life philosophy. In this modern day in which careers often take center stage, it is easy to dismiss or altogether forget our true passions. Many people work themselves to the bone either to meet basic needs or to buy that million-dollar home. The social research discussed in chapter 8 indicates that money and wealth have become passions for many young professionals. I can't tell you the number of times I have witnessed people who have spent their lives and hundreds of thousands of dollars to become MDs and PhDs struggle with their day-to-day lives simply because being an MD or a PhD was not their true passion.

Part of discovering who you are is to unlock your first principles and determine the true passions that give your life meaning.

Your Turn: Exercise 2

The objective of this exercise is to discover what you are passionate about and how you can combine that with your strengths to live in a way that gives your life meaning.

Revisit your narrative. Read through the experiences that brought you the most joy, pleasure, and meaning. Think about what drives you, what gives you purpose, what motivates you. When have you felt most alive, most in tune with your true *Self*? If you accept that loving others is what gives life meaning, how have you loved the world so far? Your answers to these questions will help lead you to the passions that will give your life meaning. As you write, you will find common themes that will uncover your passions. Write them down.

Now consider your strengths. What comes naturally to you that you enjoy doing? What can you do that no one else can do or that you do differently, better? What activities give you energy and help you perform at your personal best? Now list what you believe to be your three greatest strengths. If you have difficulty answering these questions, talk to the trusted person you shared your narrative with to help you determine what they are. Write them down.

Finally, write down how you believe you can most effectively combine your strengths with your passions. Here is an example. A friend of mine is a CPA whose passion is to teach others about finance management so they can improve their lives. In her spare time and for free, she counsels low-income individuals on the basics of budgeting and savings. In turn, this helps give meaning to her life.

I don't expect you to figure this out in a day or two. Take your time with this exercise. Once you link your passions and strengths together, you can begin to develop a specific road map that will provide your life with purpose.

I love this quote, often attributed to Oscar Wilde: "Be yourself. Everyone else is taken." It is not easy to begin the discovery process of finding your *Self*. It takes a lot of work and likely a few shed tears. But here you are, hopefully more grounded in your identity than ever before. I am so proud that you are beginning to unlock a new vision of your life. Now that you have a better idea of who you are and where you desire to go, it is time to pinpoint and call out the roadblocks that hinder you from taking that journey.

12

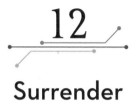

Surrender

I have been driven many times upon my knees by
the overwhelming conviction that I had no where
else to go. My own wisdom and that of all about
me seemed insufficient for that day.

Abraham Lincoln

"One day," my then-wife threatened, "I'm going to leave you."
Her words echoed in my ears. No matter how hard I tried to
convince myself otherwise, deep in my heart I knew she was
telling the truth. She would leave. I just didn't know when.

Three months later, as I drove home after a tough day
at work, my mind felt heavy, weighed down by a gnawing
premonition. When I walked through the front door of the
house we had shared for three years, my worst fears were
realized. Photos and pictures had been removed from the
walls, nails still in their lonely places. I stood shocked as

my laptop bag slipped out of my fingers and landed with a thud on the floor. I ran to the master bedroom and witnessed more evidence of my wife's abrupt departure. Her closets were empty. Dresser drawers bare. Personal items from the bathroom gone. My heart beat wildly out of my chest as I thought about my beloved stepdaughter. *One last hope.* My chest tight, I darted upstairs to her room, only to be crushed further. Clothes, books, trinkets, photos—gone.

My mind spun. I slowly made my way down the stairs and into a hallway corner. Balled up in a fetal position, I sobbed so heavily that my shoulders shook and I could barely catch my breath. I was alone. I felt lost, empty, grieved by a marriage that had finally ended so terribly.

Before you feel sorry for me, know that I deserved my fate. My ex-wife wasn't solely to blame for our failed relationship. We were both at fault. She and I were wonderful and deeply flawed people who because of our System 1 fears and insecurities in overdrive had steadily and methodically destroyed each other over the course of our relationship. To be fair, the marriage was likely doomed from the start. Not only had we both endured several highly influential and difficult childhood experiences that we had not dealt with, but we also had connected not long after the ends of destructive long-term marriages. (My first marriage had just ended as a result of similar devastating System 1 behaviors, feelings, and reactions in overdrive due to difficult pasts neither one of us had dealt with.) The combination of these factors provided the perfect recipe for a second marital disaster.

When we suffer from System 1 emotions and behaviors in overdrive, it is likely we will be attracted to others who suffer with similar issues. This results in an unhealthy fusion that eventually either demolishes the relationship or poisons us through the continual raging of civil war. These same relationship difficulties spread to the next relationship and the next and even from generation to generation until someone has the courage to stop the cycle.

Both my second ex-wife and I unknowingly transferred much from our past devastating experiences onto each other. There were times in the heat of horrible fights that we called each other by the names of significant people from our pasts. We hadn't a clue we weren't fighting each other but individually were in the midst of battles with the ghosts of yesteryears.

To be completely fair, she was not the first to walk away. Unable to deal with my own emotions and my deeply broken and undifferentiated *Self*, I had stormed out on several occasions during especially hostile arguments, staying away for days, sometimes even weeks. I refused to be vulnerable to rejection again. At times, I felt I would rather die than experience this strong childhood reaction of being unlovable, an emotion I was all too familiar with. I disappeared into my work. I thought if I put in longer hours, conducted enough life-changing research, published enough papers, got enough grants, started enough companies, and authored enough books, I would somehow become worthy of love and all the bad stuff would magically go away.

In case you are wondering, prior to her departure, my wife and I spent a year seeing three Christian counselors (one for me, one for her, and one for the both of us) in hopes of saving our marriage. Many of our counseling sessions focused on our feelings and the anatomy of our fights. In hindsight, with all due respect to these therapists, these things did not matter and remedying them could not save our marriage.

The problem lay in our individual pasts. We had to recognize that our feelings toward each other were simply System 1 emotions, illusions, echoes, and repercussions from previous experiences that were being redirected toward each other. Unfortunately, we weren't provided that message.

In the following illustration (Figure 12.1), notice that in an unhealthy relationship, the two people try to shoot arrows at their problems, but because fear, transference, parental attachments, and other experiences stand between them, they end up shooting arrows at each other. By contrast, in a healthy relationship, the two people are allies in shooting arrows at their problems, not at each other. Tragically, my ex-wife and I were like the first couple.

Figure 12.1

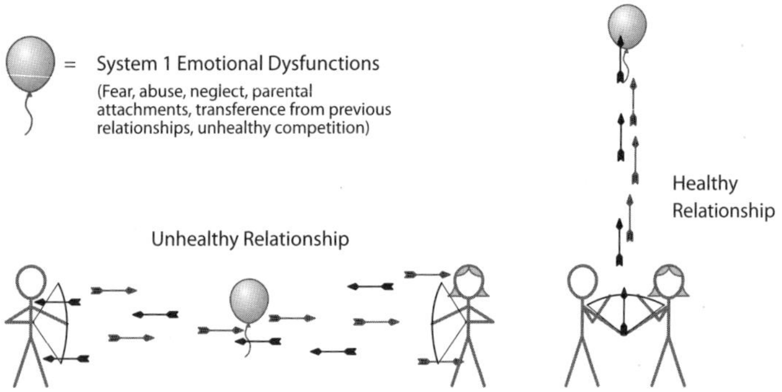

= System 1 Emotional Dysfunctions
(Fear, abuse, neglect, parental attachments, transference from previous relationships, unhealthy competition)

Healthy Relationship

Unhealthy Relationship

Rock Bottom: The Bedrock of Change

Much of the last two years of my second marriage was tough, to put it mildly. My health deteriorated dramatically. I was on antidepressants and high blood pressure medication. I was also dealing with the early stages of the same aggressive form of prostate cancer that had killed my father.

I was an emotional wreck, devastated by overwhelming guilt, shame, and embarrassment at the growing disconnect and strife between my then-wife and me. Though I had always dreamed of having a godly marriage that would last forever, I was helping bring to ruins the one thing that I cared about the most and deeply wounding our children in the process. Not only was I failing my family, but I was also letting down my spiritual community. While I had been in leadership roles in both the Presbyterian and Methodist churches and knew and constantly studied the Bible and works of greats like C. S. Lewis, Mother Teresa, and Dietrich Bonhoeffer, I couldn't keep a family together. What hurt most, however, was the thought that I had disappointed God. Though I loved him with all my heart, soul, and mind, I feared I had fallen from his grace.

As illogical as this sounds to me today, a few months before my ex-wife actually left me, I also started to believe that my failures and sins had caused all the tragedies in my life, including the automobile accident and subsequent paralysis of my son Josh. This thought was particularly frightening because it had the potential to completely destroy me. I could tackle the guilt from the bad decisions that had led to the failure of my first marriage and what seemed like an inevitable second divorce. I could also reasonably accept that somehow in a balanced universe my mistakes had led to my cancer diagnosis. But I could not handle being responsible for my son's calamity. Had the consequences of my sins fallen on my child? If this was true, I couldn't bear to live.

This was my bottom.

Rock bottom as it concerns alcoholism is "the place an alcoholic must reach before he finally is ready to admit that he has a problem and reaches out for help."[1] It may be the fifth DUI, waking up facedown on a sidewalk in an unfamiliar city and having no clue how you got there, losing custody of your children, or simply being sick and tired of being sick and tired. While rock bottom in addiction looks different for everyone, it is often visible and definable. And it is typically the catalyst for change.

Unfortunately, because we have little understanding of and few support systems for people who suffer from emotional dysfunctions as a result of System 1 in overdrive, finding the bottom and climbing your way out of the hole are harder to articulate. This is a major reason why I have written this book and particularly this chapter—to help others sense where they are in their emotional battles and what the bottom can look like for someone with System 1 dysfunctions. This understanding ultimately paves the pathway to transformation.

When you can name, can admit to, and are ready and committed to remedy your System 1 emotional dysfunctions, you are at the foot of the hill of change. As this book draws to an end, I am confident you are close. You have come far. You have begun to look deep within your *Self* and acknowledge your trouble spots. You may be aware of the particular emotional dysfunctions from System 1 in overdrive that plague you and abort positive forward movement. Or you may need more help. If this is you, the following exercise will help you name your emotional dysfunction.

Your Turn

In the previous chapter, the exploratory exercises focused on discovering who you are, the story of your life, what you are most passionate about, and what gives your life meaning and joy. Now it is time to take the difficult journey of uncovering the System 1 dysfunctions that have prevented you from expressing your true *Self*.

Revisit the story you wrote in the previous chapter. You may have had great difficulty living out your passions and finding meaning in your life. Much of this incapacity is likely due to past events and relationships that have led to magnified fears, transference and attachment issues, and other dysfunctions. After reading through this book, answering the questions at the end of each chapter, and writing your *Self*-narrative, you probably have an idea of what System 1 in overdrive looks like in your life. Now it is time to call out specific issues. In this exercise, your System 2 is on a quest to uncover the System 1 mega-superhighway in your mind.

1. Begin with prayer. Ask God to help reveal negative patterns and behaviors that are detrimental to your well-being and *Self*-expression.

2. Name your emotional dysfunction(s). You have likely experienced difficult, stressful, or even traumatic experiences growing up or even as an adult that have impacted you in a significant and particularly negative way. What are the most critical relationships you have had that have affected your life the most and produced internal and external conflict? How have these experiences affected your relationships with others and your overall quality of life? For example, perhaps you endured emotional, physical, or another form of abuse or neglect from a parent and now you unconsciously transfer those emotions onto your significant other. Maybe you or someone

you loved suffered through a trauma that produced in you a driving need to control or excessive fear that has sucked the joy out of life. Maybe you have difficulty forgiving others, or you are easily frustrated by small things that block your goals, or sadness pervades your life, or you are inclined to judge others negatively, or you are *Self*-critical to an excessive degree, or you are easily jealous, or you avoid people and situations that might expose you to rejection. These are just a few of the many possible emotional dysfunctions.

3. Based on what you have written above, have you hit an emotional rock bottom or are you heading toward one? Alternatively, are you simply existing, living in a difficult dream world but never really waking up, taking a slow but torturous journey down a well-trodden road that will likely end with regrets? Are you willing to do something about this to change the trajectory of your life?

4. Share this part of your story with the same person who read the first part in the previous chapter. Ask this person for feedback. Is your view of your emotional dysfunctions consistent with how this person interprets your experience and your life?

5. This exercise may be particularly emotional for you and may dredge up anxiety, sadness, or anger. If necessary, meet with a counselor or professional spiritual advisor to explore and work through these issues.

Now that you have a new conceptual framework for your emotional dysfunctions, it is time to change. *Self*-exploratory work is essentially useless unless you use that information to begin the transformation process.

The Underlying Neuroscience behind Change

Change is not an event; it is a process. In chapter 4, I compared the brain science of our System 1 emotions and behaviors to the busiest highway in the United States, the fourteen-lane I-405, and brain plasticity to the fictional highway construction company Neurogenesis. As a result of my negative childhood events, I developed a highway of brain circuitry surrounding my System 1 fears of not being worthy or lovable. As I experienced rejection and similar painful events later in life, that highway became larger and stronger. Over the course of my life, specifically in repeating System 1 fight-or-flight behaviors in my relationships, I was unconsciously building even larger mega-superhighways associated with abandonment, rejection, and fear. When I began the process of surrendering my emotional dysfunctions, which I will talk about in a bit, it was time to deconstruct old mega-superhighways and create new ones.

I believe surrendering your System 1 dysfunctions, your old way of living and thinking, to God—or a higher power, to use the language of Alcoholics Anonymous—provides the critical mechanism that makes brain rewiring possible. This process enables your unconscious to pay less attention to distressful feelings and behaviors because it "knows" you have given them to God. This reduces the number of nerve impulses that move along established System 1 mega-superhighways in your mind. Remember, the golden rule of brain plasticity is that the circuits or highways used most get stronger and those not used get weaker and eventually deteriorate. Surrender opens your *Self*, your mind, to the possibility of building new circuits to well-being. In the illustration in chapter 4 of a balanced System 1 and 2 response, recall that surrender is shown as the jackhammer operator breaking up the extra lanes of System 1.

At first, change is very difficult. Your mind still wants to use the mega-superhighways it is familiar with, no matter how emotionally destructive they are. However, when you give up these highways to God and choose with your System 2 reasoning to use new roads through daily practices (I will share a few of these), newly formed roads begin to rapidly expand into two-lane highways. With continued usage, they eventually transform into mega-superhighways that if continually traveled will lead toward a destination of peace, joy, contentment, and wholeness.

You can see how surrender sits at the epicenter of any life-altering transformation. You cannot simply will your *Self* to stop damaging habits and tendencies that arise in your unconscious. Control is your enemy! Don't believe me? Just see what happens when you try to change by continuing to control your thoughts, actions, and behaviors with your own will. You are simply using the same mega-superhighways that got you in trouble to begin with.

Perhaps you have said something like, "Tomorrow I'll start being more patient with my kids and will never scream at them again." Or "This is the last time I mess around with another woman on a business trip." Or "I'm giving up smoking for good this time." In saying these words and white-knuckling the process, you are fully confident that your desire to change is strong enough to make it happen. Unfortunately, this is misguided confidence. Control cannot coexist with surrender; on the contrary, it is a saboteur. You might as well stand in the middle of the heavily trafficked I-405 waving your arms and screaming at every moving vehicle to stop and expecting them to do so. Remember, millions of nerve signals per day travel on the System 1 superhighways of your brain. Your conscious will alone cannot stop this rushing influx of unconscious thoughts, memories, emotions, and sensations. You will get run over every time.

A System 2–Led Transformation

Transformation requires a conscious System 2 decision and unbending commitment for your life to be different, better. I have broken this process down into five simple steps. I am confident that this far into the book you have conquered the first three.

Step 1. Admit that the way you have lived in many of the most important areas of your life has not worked for you, specifically in being driven by System 1 emotional dysfunctions.

Step 2. Make a determined System 2 choice that you are no longer willing to continue to approach life using the same System 1 behaviors and emotions that you have depended on in the past. You must also understand that this journey of change is difficult and will take considerable time.

Step 3. Surrender your emotional dysfunctions—your old patterns, thinking, and behaviors—to God. What does this mean? Initially, it is as simple as praying this commitment aloud in your own words and with conviction. Ask God for help during this process. If prayer does not come easily to you, use the following model taken from St. Ignatius:

Take, Lord, and receive all my liberty,
my memory, my understanding
and my entire will,
All I have and call my own.
You have given all to me.
To you, Lord, I return it.
Everything is yours; do with it what you will.
Give me only your love and your grace.
That is enough for me.[2]

Remember, just because you prayed a prayer of surrender does not mean you won't be tempted to retake control. Change takes time. Surrender in this context is making official your commitment to let go of what has been holding you back. You will need to continue surrendering your emotional dysfunctions every day, sometimes even several times a day, as you work through your issues.

Step 4. Once you say yes to the process of surrender, it is time to build a new life, beginning with constructing new mega-superhighways that will give your life meaning and joy. This course will include a great deal of contemplative prayer and meditation as you deepen your insight into your *Self* and your journey. This is not a journey to take alone. You are a co-creator with God of a new life. You must do your part. In chapter 4, I reminded you that your own thoughts are your most powerful weapons for transformation. With God's guidance, you now must build new superhighways by telling your *Self* a new story about how your life will be. "For as he [a man or woman] thinks within himself, so he is" (Prov. 23:7 NASB).

Step 5. Find a counselor, professional spiritual advisor, mentor, or support group to guide you on this difficult journey of change. This is critical. I want to be clear that some of the emotional dysfunctions you suffer from cannot be rewired simply by reading this book. Get the help you need going forward.

My Surrender

After hitting bottom and refusing to continue living with inconsistencies, I cried out to God in prayer. I simply told him, "I give up! Please help me!" This was my genesis of surrender. I also started a series of intense counseling sessions with Frank Seekins, an internationally recognized Hebrew biblical scholar and marriage counselor. Like Angel Second Class Clarence in the movie *It's a Wonderful Life*, my therapist was a very unlikely character. I had never met him, and because he lived on the other side of the country, our sessions were conducted over the telephone. I don't even remember how I found him. I believe it was through a friend's recommendation, but I am just not sure.

Frank mentored me several times a week for six months, starting three months before I arrived at my empty home that night. Unlike Clarence, Frank did not show me all the wonderful things I had done in my life but instead helped me to understand how broken I was. His first order of business was to reveal the ways that my brain wiring and resulting thinking patterns were wrong when it came to how I approached relationships. He made it clear that I was doomed to repeat the same mistakes over and over again if I did not surrender my emotional strongholds, particularly my desperate need to control and my overwhelming fear of being rejected and abandoned. Frank also pointed out from the beginning of our time together that my marriage was so deeply maimed that reconciliation was unlikely. However, he was confident that God could use even that wreckage and my inconsolable pain to transform my *Self*.

He was right.

Frank taught me that surrender is turning away from what has taken control over you and gaining something of greater value. In Hebrew, the word *surrender* means "to bow the knee." For me, this means having absolute confidence in Jesus's words, "Come to me, all of you who are weary and carry heavy burdens, and I will give you rest. Take my yoke upon you. Let me teach you, because I am humble and gentle at heart, and you will find rest for your souls" (Matt. 11:28–29 NLT).

Notice Christ's requirement in this verse: "Take my yoke upon you." A yoke is "a wooden crosspiece that is fastened over the necks of two animals and attached to the plow or cart that they are to pull."[3] When I was growing up in the country, our family used a 1957 Massey Ferguson tractor to plow our fields, but some of my neighbors still employed oxen. I remember the theatrics showcased by the younger animals when the farmhands would fasten the yoke on them for the first time. If one was particularly spirited and independent, it would go crazy trying to attack the wooden crosspiece, the other ox, or anyone or anything else nearby. Eventually, however, the animal would settle down and surrender to the yoke. Otherwise, it would become hamburger meat.

When I started talking to Frank, a part of me was like a feisty ox, not completely ready or willing to give up control.

Consequently, the yoke of surrender still had a lot of pain in store for me. But that is the price of being rewired. And that is why it is not easy and takes time. My goal in the process of surrendering was to one day live in peace and freedom and be able to manage well my feelings of fear, anxiety, guilt, and shame to maintain healthy relationships. I have mentioned that alcoholics in the beginning stages of recovery are advised to weather the process one day (and sometimes one minute) at a time. This is how I approached the pathway of surrender.

Practices That Lead to Rewiring

I have already offered five steps that fuel the process of transformation. I would like to add four practices that Frank suggested that helped me break free from the bondage of emotional dysfunctions (these work in conjunction with the aforementioned steps). I can say with confidence this advice helped me not only recognize and learn how to handle my emotional strongholds but also discover, define, and love my *Self*.

Pray—all the time. Prayer became a discipline not as a channel to ask God to help save my marriage but as a means to develop a personal relationship with him. Simply talking to God regularly as I would a trusted friend helped me on a daily basis to surrender my pain, my confusion, and my will. I was amazed at how over time my prayers morphed from selfish monologues to quiet times of meditation as I simply asked God to guide me in this process and uncover my true *Self*. Whatever your spiritual background, prayer is important. It is a critical component to the process of surrender, an admission that you desperately need help outside of your *Self*.

Take responsibility for your part. No matter how strongly I believed I was standing on moral high ground in my marriage, the fact was I was not. I was a major contributor to the problems. I had not acted well, led well, or exemplified how to love well, and for that I was ultimately responsible. Consequently, I needed to apologize for the state of the marriage and in the process surrender my need to be right. It didn't matter if my wife accepted my apologies or returned my words with hostility. I simply had to say I was sorry. When we admit we are wrong and become accountable for our actions, we open the door to healing. It is another way of telling the universe we are ready to embrace change.

Be vulnerable. I would have to do the one thing I feared the most: make my *Self* vulnerable. Ironically, doing so opened the door to my ultimate liberation. After much prayer and contemplation, I felt God leading me to tell my wife "I love you" three times each day until the marriage was either repaired or over. I started three months before she left and did this from the bottom of my heart, absent of expectation. God was teaching me about true love, giving my *Self* without expecting anything in return. If I was to love in that manner, I had to trust that he would give me so much more love in return, that his love was more than enough. When you trust in God, in his provision, in his plan, and in his timing, you are better able to open your *Self* in humility to others. You tend to do the right thing regardless of the outcome.

Spend time in solitude to Self-*reflect*. Frank asked that outside of work and spending time with my four children and new granddaughter, I stay home for five months, even on the weekends. He wasn't being a killjoy; he just wanted me to, for the first time in my life, face my *Self*. No distractions.

No opportunities to escape or numb my *Self* at cocktail parties or get-togethers.

I used that time to pray, meditate, and *Self*-reflect. Being alone was difficult at first, but the more time that passed, the more I learned to love and take care of my *Self*. I will admit Frank paid a heavy price for this directive. At first, I suffered panic attacks and was convinced I would go crazy without some form of live social stimulation. I can't tell you how many 3:00 a.m. phone calls we shared over my fear that I would not be able to continue this practice of contemplative solitude.

We live in a society in which no one wants to be alone. We are glued to our technologic devices and addicted to social media, which, as discussed in chapter 5, serve to suppress the ache of loneliness that defines the human condition. But intentionally getting in touch with your *Self* is critical. You learn how to soothe your *Self*. You come face-to-face with certain realities that have been clouded by distraction. You become more attuned to your emotional and mental structure as you move through the process of change. You fuel your momentum to keep going.

Change, Eventually

Lest you think I put these practices into action immediately, and with ease and without slipups, know I did not. During my time with Frank, I continued to make some critical mistakes. For instance, I engaged in a few destructive emotional outbursts aimed at my wife that I am not proud of. Each time when I felt I had failed, Frank reminded me that it was not possible for me to change in a few weeks. Rewiring our minds takes months, even years. When you fall back on your old patterns or behaviors, know that you have not failed. Look at these setbacks as opportunities to pause, recognize your mistake, and do things better the next time. Human beings aren't perfect, and our emotions are real. As we move through painful transitions, scars run deep. It takes time to learn and grow and progress into a stable, strong, and flexible *Self*.

The most amazing part of my journey is that daily weaving in the four practices ultimately helped me rewire my mind in the midst of incredible pain and anxiety. It was at this point that I began to read and study everything I could find in biology, psychology, and philosophy journals and textbooks concerning the underpinnings of dual process reasoning. The book you are holding in your hand right now is the result of that tremendous learning journey. Who knew the road I would travel after struggling through the aftermath of such destruction? Miracles do exist, indeed!

Relax, God's Got This

A. W. Tozer wrote, "The reason why many are still troubled, still seeking, still making little forward progress is because they haven't yet come to the end of themselves. We're still trying to give orders, and interfering with God's work within us."[4]

As a *Self*-proclaimed recovering control freak, I am still learning how to engage life with love as it comes and not how I orchestrated it. Instead of trying desperately to control my situation or others', I have surrendered this control and have chosen to go with the flow. I now try every day to reply to the universe with love, and I have given up my insistence that the universe respond to me. This doesn't mean I am a bystander in life, spending my days locked away in meditation chanting the mantra "Que sera sera." On the contrary, I engage in life and in relationships and aim to make a difference in whatever I do. The difference in my life today since my rock bottom is my unwavering trust in God—being settled in my spirit by the fact that he leads and guides me, even through the circumstances in which I have no control. I understand that I cannot change others or dictate how they relate or respond to me. I acknowledge the occasional temptation to want to help God manage his role and will in my life, but at my core I know that his way is always better. As I always say, "God's got this." Boy, does that take the pressure off!

Life isn't easy. We suffer bruises, scrapes, and deep cuts that beckon us to give up and live on the sidelines, imprisoned by our fears. If this is you, look within and you will find a glimpse of a brave soul. Understand that life is wrought with the unpredictable. Risks, confusion, and pain abound. But walking through them consciously, aware, and open will lead to a life full of meaning, passion, and well-being. You are not alone. God is with you as you journey through change step by step. And though the road is long, as your mind rewires itself, hope resurrects. Life gets better and brighter and you begin to see the handprint of God, of love, all around. Trust me, he's got this.

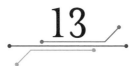

13

Forgiveness and Freedom

We must develop and maintain the capacity to forgive. He who is devoid of the power to forgive is devoid of the power to love. There is some good in the worst of us and some evil in the best of us. When we discover this, we are less prone to hate our enemies.

Martin Luther King Jr.

As I write this chapter, just three days ago, a deeply troubled twenty-one-year-old young man walked into a historic African American church in Charleston, South Carolina. A .45 caliber handgun was hidden in his fanny pack. For one hour, this young man sat in a pew during an ongoing Bible study. And then he opened fire, uttering words of racial hatred and killing nine people in that sanctuary. The death of these saints, six women and three men, left thousands of families and friends and a nation in mourning. And while this tragic shooting occurred during a time of ongoing racial unrest and divide in which retribution for injustice demanded more blood spilled, more violence, more chaos, and more rage, something peculiar happened in Charleston.

Family members of the victims reached out to the shooter not with press conferences or hatred but with great sadness and, remarkably, forgiveness. During a bond hearing held days after the mass murder, these relatives were allowed to address the defendant in court via video.

A woman whose mother was killed said, "You took something very precious away from me. I will never talk to her ever again. I will never be able to hold her again. But I forgive you. And have mercy on your soul."[1]

A sister of another victim said, "I acknowledge that I am very angry, but she [her sister] taught me that we are the family that love built. We have no room for hating."[2] The capacity of these beautiful souls to forgive just days after their losses reminds us that there is a way to address evil that does not involve hate or retribution: the powerful act of forgiveness.

This brings to mind another tragic shooting that took place in an Amish schoolhouse in 2006. A truck driver stormed a peaceful community in Pennsylvania, killing five girls and injuring five others before turning his weapon on himself. With an unfathomable grace and compassion, the Amish people reached out to the murderer's wife and family. A grandfather of one of the victims made this shocking statement: "We must not think evil of this man."[3] Another member of the community said, "I don't think there's anybody here that wants to do anything but forgive and not only reach out to those who have suffered a loss in that way but to reach out

to the family of the man who committed these acts."⁴ Several
of the victims' parents even attended the shooter's funeral,
embracing the grieving widow he left behind.
Forgiveness is a powerful force. To our System 1 animal
nature, it is illogical, irrational, and simply makes no sense.
System 1 is a danger warning system that insists we always
remember and whenever possible take action to eliminate
a threat and anyone associated with it. Perhaps this is why
forgiveness is truly an impetus of transformation that brings
light from darkness, freedom from the atrocities of our past,
and endless potential for peace in each moment and the
future.

Forgiving Others

Throughout this book, I have emphasized the importance
of being honest with your *Self*. Doing so allows you to take
responsibility for your actions and surrender your will to
God. While this is an important process in rewiring your
mind, the next step is forgiveness, forgiving others (and your
Self) who have caused you pain.
Forgiveness is essential for a healthy soul, mind, and body.
Psychologist Robert Enright, author of several books, including *The Forgiving Life*, said in a recent interview that through
the act of forgiving "people can expect lower anxiety, lower
anger, lower depression if there is any, and a greater sense
of self-esteem and hopefulness and healthier relationships
because you are not bringing those wounds into your relationships with others."⁵
Even as I write these words, I admit I can't imagine the
horror you may have endured. While I have laid bare my story,

you may have experienced utter evil. During my counseling sessions, Frank taught me the difference between sin and evil. He said the word *sin*, as used in the Bible, has several Hebrew roots and meanings, but the one I should apply to my situation and my life was "missing the mark or target." As you already know, for a long time I felt guilty for being a terrible person who perpetrated a relational catastrophe, even to the point of attributing the awful tragedies in my life to my actions. Frank offered that the biblical use of the word *evil* was making a choice to carry out an action that would intentionally hurt others. This was not the case in my relationships. God knew my heart, and though I had made misguided and detrimental mistakes, I would never intentionally hurt another. Understanding that critical concept helped me to forgive my *Self*.

It is easier to forgive a person for missing the mark than for committing an evil act; still, even in light of senseless atrocities, forgiveness is necessary for one's well-being. So how does one forgive evil? And what does that mean? I want to be clear that forgiving others does not minimize or deny what others have done to hurt you. It is about releasing unhealthy emotions such as resentment and bitterness and the weight of being victimized so you can experience personal freedom. It is critical to remember the words of artist and author C. R. Strahan: "Forgiveness has nothing to do with absolving a criminal of his crime. It has everything to do with relieving oneself of the burden of being a victim—letting go of the pain and transforming oneself from victim to survivor."[6]

I know of a circumstance in which a father raped one of his young daughters for years at the same time he was sexually abusing other neighborhood children. Forgiveness in this type of abusive situation will necessitate boundaries. In the case of the girl, who is now a grown woman with a family of her own, though she has forgiven her father, she has also rightfully chosen never to see him again. Even under horrific circumstances, forgiveness should not be viewed as a liability but as a *Self*-loving and powerful pathway to freedom.

Forgiveness calls for a deep understanding of Martin Luther King Jr.'s words that "there is some good in the worst of us and some evil in the best of us." As we recognize our imperfections and pay attention to the destructive nature of some of our own thoughts and immoral actions, forgiving others becomes doable. It is critical to acknowledge this principle because rather than admit to our flaws, mistakes, or character failures, our natural tendency is to initially address these shortcomings with excuses and rationalizations that protect our integrity. This prevents us from seeing our failings for what they really are. Ironically, we often do just the opposite with those who hurt us, inflating their failings. Underestimating our possible responsibility in an area of intense conflict or tension increases the chance that we overestimate the role of another. So we become and remain the victim.

A good example is when a marriage dissolves. How many messy divorces have you witnessed? Perhaps you have been through one of your own. In these situations, two people, along with their families, friends, and attorneys, carry out legal and PR offensives to discredit and destroy each other. This is the human reptilian brain in attack mode. One of my good friends is a divorce attorney, and he told me a common expression used in his profession: "We eat what we kill."

Ironically, when spouses seek to annihilate each other financially, mentally, or emotionally with every System 1 competitive and survival instinct imaginable, the only people who win these vicious fighting matches are the lawyers.

Dr. King has always been a hero of mine, but my respect for him recently grew as I revisited and dissected his writings and sermons. In his famous "Loving Your Enemies" message delivered in Montgomery, Alabama, in 1957, King preached on Jesus's commandment to love our enemies (see Matt. 5:44). The civil rights activist emphasized how hate, along with the accompanying emotions of pride, jealousy, anger, and resentment, is the driving force behind unforgiveness. He posited that it is only by truly and courageously loving that we are able to forgive. This in turn frees us from hate and all the unruly and suffocating refuse that tags along with it. (Keep in mind King made a distinction between love and like. We can love people we don't necessarily have to like.)

Two quotations from this incredible sermon have deep personal and philosophical significance to me. The first is:

> Forgiveness does not mean ignoring what has been done or putting a false label on an evil act. It means, rather, that the evil act no longer remains a barrier to the relationship. Forgiveness is a catalyst creating the atmosphere necessary for a fresh start and a new beginning. It is the lifting of a burden or the cancelation of a debt.[7]

Jesus once told a parable about a king who forgave his servant by canceling an owed debt and releasing him from all financial obligations (see Matt. 18:23–35). King offered that this act is the critical first step to a fresh new start for the individual who forgives as well as the forgiven. While reconciliation is not always possible, forgiving another does provide an opportunity for a new beginning that may not have otherwise existed.

The second quotation is by far the most famous. I believe these are among the most important words spoken in my lifetime: "Darkness cannot drive out darkness; only light can do that. Hate cannot drive out hate; only love can do that."[8] Do you want to know the key to freedom on this earth? It is this extraordinary System 2 principle of not returning hate with hate but responding to hate with love.

It is the moving comeback of the beautiful community of Charleston's Emanuel African Methodist Episcopal Church when evil pillaged its sanctuary. It is the whispered sentiment of the Amish people when innocent children were gunned down. It is what you and I have the capacity to do, though it is certainly not easy, seems unnatural, and defies logic. It is an act of heroism, evidencing Christlike compassion and mercy.

Our System 1 survival instincts clearly convey just the opposite. They tell us to attack or run from anyone who is a threat. Jesus's call to love our enemies and King's emphasis on this teaching ask us to go against everything that is innately wired into the primitive portions of our brains. This requires a profoundly differentiated *Self* and extensive rewiring.

In his recent book *Forgiveness Is Living*, supported by decades of research, Robert Enright describes how forgiveness heals and can be used to improve health and suffering. He and others write about how forgiveness is a process that can become a habit when you do the following:

- First, examine how injustice affects your emotions (like anger, hate, and bitterness). Overwhelming negative thoughts and emotions and feeling powerless can be great motivators for change to regain your power.

- Second, decide to change your inner world that has been damaged by injustice. As you learn and practice forgiveness, you offer your *Self* peace, mercy, and goodness.
- Third, know that you do not need to condone evil or excuse or reconcile with your offender or abuser, especially if it is not safe to do so.[9]

In the next several pages, you will have the opportunity to address unforgiveness in your heart and explore whether or not it is a stronghold. But first, it is important to explore another facet of this issue.

Forgiving Your *Self*

Perhaps what is harder than forgiving others is staring at our own reflection in the mirror and having to offer that same grace. For many, showing compassion and kindness to themselves is wrought with guilt and shame, paralyzing forward movement.

A friend of mine told me a powerful and tragic story about what happened to her family over fifty years ago. Ten brothers and sisters grew up in a small, rural farming community where they settled as adults and raised their own families. Hunting was a necessary and common practice; accidents, unfortunately, were prevalent. One day, a son of one of the sisters headed out with his best friend and his cousin to find and shoot a deer for dinner. Tragically, the young boy mistook his cousin for their intended prey and accidently shot and killed him. Overwhelmed by guilt, he refused to forgive himself, even when this boy's aunt, the mother of the victim, pleaded with the lad to find it in his heart to forgive himself, as she had forgiven him for what was a terrible accident.

Years went by. As the boy became a man, his *Self*-hatred and shame grew stronger. He felt indebted to his aunt and out of guilt constantly asked to do chores for her. The woman assured him she needed nothing from him save for his *Self*-forgiveness. But no matter how hard she tried to console her nephew, he was unable to grant himself the same mercy she had shown him. This man died at a young age, alone, broken, and deeply disturbed.

One of the most troubling aspects of this story is the sweeping impact of this man's inability to forgive himself; it affected the rest of his extended family. No one ever dared speak of the boy who died because it would inevitably bring to the surface the one who had accidentally killed him. Because this family was unable to celebrate the lives of the two deceased, their capacity to grieve was truncated. For years following the accident, it was only mentioned behind closed doors and in secretive whispers, usually when an unsuspecting younger family member broached the topic.

Our inability to forgive our *Selves* affects others, even for generations to come. I have recently said to my ex-wife that while we may not have shown our children how to love well, we can show and have shown them how to forgive properly.

The act of forgiving your *Self* is difficult when you are being choked by the suffocating clutches of guilt and shame. There is a distinction between the two. Guilt is often appropriate. It occurs when we realize we have fallen short of our personal values and God's morality. This realization should be uncomfortable enough that it motivates us toward true change. Guilt is not necessarily a bad thing as long as it doesn't fester and morph into shame.

Bestselling author Brené Brown makes a clear distinction between guilt and shame:

> A clear way to see the difference is to think about this question: If you made a mistake that really hurt someone's feelings, would you be willing to say, "I'm sorry. I made a mistake"? If you're experiencing guilt, the answer is yes: "I *made* a mistake." Shame, on the other hand, is, "I'm sorry. I *am* a mistake." Shame doesn't just sound different than guilt; it feels different. Once we understand this distinction, guilt can even make us feel more positively about ourselves, because it points to the gap between what we did and who we are—and, thankfully, we can change what we do.[10]

During the time I felt trapped by shame, feeling responsible for my son's accident because of my moral failings, I will never forget what happened to help shift my perspective. On a particularly bad day, I went for a drive. I sped down the highway, weeping uncontrollably. I heard my cell phone ring and ignored the call. But the phone kept ringing incessantly. Not paying attention to the caller's name flashing on the screen, I finally picked up the phone. Before slamming it down on the passenger seat, I yelled into the speaker, "Leave me alone!"

No such luck. Another incoming call. Realizing it was my younger sister Tanya, I sighed and answered the phone. Tanya and I love each other dearly, but truth be told, we have been fighting since the day she was born.

I was sobbing so hard it was hard to talk. My sister ordered me to pull off to the side of the road. She scolded, "Don't you understand that you could cause a wreck and kill someone in such a crazy emotional state?"

After following her instruction and taking a minute to catch my breath and settle down, I expressed my feelings of shame. I even told her that if I was, in fact, the reason my son had to suffer, I wanted to die.

While Tanya had no words of sympathy for her distraught older brother, she did offer wisdom in the form of tough love. "Would you hush for a minute?" she began, then paused before continuing in a rather harsh tone. "You're just a big old fake, aren't you, Ski? You don't believe a thing you have been taught in Sunday school and church all these years."

"What do you mean?" I asked.

"Ski, you get a new slate every day. As long as you are sorry and have asked for forgiveness for the previous day's sins, God has forgiven and forgotten them. Any dummy knows that. You got a clean slate yesterday, and the day before, and the day before that. So Josh's accident could not have been your fault. What on earth is wrong with you? You know full well that grace is the centerpiece of our faith. It's the only way any of us can really be free!"

My baby sister was right. How could I have missed that?

If you have been beating your *Self* up for something you did years ago, or even recently, but have taken responsibility for your actions, it is time to stop. It is time to heal. *Self*-forgiveness is essential for you to get unstuck. You can't change the past, but you can change the trajectory of your life going forward.

Your Turn

Forgiveness is a deeply profound experience that will allow you to take back your power and joy. It is worth it, especially when you share and help others through your experience. Take some time and reflect on the current state of your life.

Revisit the *Self*-narrative you wrote in chapter 11. Can you pinpoint certain characteristics (such as anger, strained relationships, negativity) that might result from not fully forgiving past hurts? Perhaps you are unable to maintain healthy relationships because you are harboring a deep resentment against a family member for abusing you growing up. Maybe you won't allow your *Self* to be happy or have fun because of the tremendous shame you feel from something you did. Unforgiveness might be your biggest stumbling block to being free. The following exercise will help you begin the rewiring process to disconnect you from the emotional dysfunctions that plague you because of unforgiveness.

Before you begin, if this area has been your biggest roadblock to living a better life, I highly recommend you seek counseling in a safe environment to work through this issue. Though this exercise is a great start, you may need more guidance than I can offer in one chapter of a book.

Begin by doing the following:

1. Write down the names of all who have caused you pain or harm that you have difficulty forgiving.
2. Write down the offenses committed against you and how you feel about them. Don't hold back.
3. Write down what has held you back from forgiving them and why it is important to forgive.

4. Now take some time to reflect, meditate, and pray to God for help to forgive these people. Remember, this doesn't mean you absolve their guilt or minimize the offense. You are simply opening the door in your heart to freedom.

5. It may also be helpful to share this exercise with a trusted friend, professional spiritual advisor, or mentor with whom you feel safe.

If your struggle resides in *Self*-forgiveness, do the following:

1. Bring to mind areas in your life or events where you have caused your *Self* or others pain, hurt, or harm.

2. If you have taken responsibility for your actions but continue to experience guilt and shame, write down how these overpowering emotions have affected your life and your relationships with others.

3. In prayer, humbly ask God to forgive you for your mistakes and moral failings that have hurt others. Through reflection and meditation, offer forgiveness and grace to your *Self*. Affirm this action with positive statements such as "I forgive my *Self*," even if you don't feel like it. Remember, forgiveness is not an emotion. It is a choice. You may not be flooded with warmth and fuzzies as you forgive others or your *Self*, but you are still making a powerful choice to free your *Self* and create an inner sanctuary of peace, health, and joy.

4. If you have not yet done so, it is important to apologize to and make amends with those you have hurt wherever possible, except when to do so would cause more damage. Saying "I'm sorry" has been a very important part

of my journey. I have not always received immediate forgiveness, but this has allowed me to complete my part of the forgiveness journey.

The Power of Freedom

Forgiveness holds the capacity to powerfully transform our *Selves* and release freedom in our lives. Through this life-giving channel, we are freed from the chains of our hang-ups, our hurts, our insecurities, our guilt, and our shame. We are free to love. We are free to enjoy life.

Freedom is such an essential, beautiful, and unique aspect of human existence. C. S. Lewis said of freedom that

> though it makes evil possible, is also the only thing that makes possible any love or goodness or joy worth having. A world of automata—of creatures that worked like machines—would hardly be worth creating. The happiness which God designs for His higher creatures is the happiness of being freely, voluntarily united to Him and to each other in an ecstasy of love and delight compared with which the most rapturous love between a man and a woman on this earth is mere milk and water. And for that they've got to be free.[11]

I believe God bet everything on our freedom. When he created us, he knew that we, with these primitive System 1 brains, would use that freedom to devastate ourselves and others. He knew that unless he attached puppet strings or surrounded us with a containment fence we would tear each other apart. And he would witness the abuse of that freedom in the form of mass murders, genocide, racism, sexual and emotional abuse, neglect, destroyed marriages, broken families, and addiction. Freedom has exacted and continues to exact an incredibly heavy price on humanity. But to God, it is worth it. Why?

Love and freedom are the most defining concepts of human existence. Though they carry separate meanings, they are not independent of each other; they are deeply interconnected. Each word gives the other meaning. Freedom cradles the potential to choose love—the unfathomable and unexplainable love that prompts a teenage son from Charleston to forgive the young man who killed his mother; or that compels a woman to forgive her father for sexually abusing her throughout her childhood and adolescence and, in his old age, to take care of him financially and in other ways; or that influences parents of an anti-apartheid activist in South Africa who was brutally murdered by black Cape Town residents to forgive their daughter's killers and set up a nonprofit organization to help South African youth.

The Freedom to Change

While writing this book, I experienced a particularly beautiful Easter morning that helped me understand our desperate need for forgiveness and Easter. I took time later that morning to write about my experience:

> In my hurry to get started this morning, I forget that today is Sunday. Then suddenly I realize that it's not just any Sunday; it's Easter Sunday. I sit at the kitchen table looking out my window as dawn peeks lazily above the horizon. My phone tells me the sun will rise in nine minutes, enough time for me to grab a coat, warm my coffee, and run outside to my backyard to behold the morning's glory.

As I shiver in the dawn chill, my eyes rest on the magnificent orange sky stretched low and speckled with bold hues of yellow and red. Staring at the bursts of color, I realize I am not wearing shoes. And I'm freezing sitting outside on this early April morning blanketed by 37 degrees of cold. Then the chill dissipates. My attention is drawn toward the first brilliant rays of light as the sun begins to rise. A new day. A new dawn. Easter Sunday.

My sunrise rendezvous reminds me that Easter, the day on the Christian calendar when we celebrate the resurrection of Christ, signifies that we are free. Free from sin, yes, but it embodies so much more. Easter symbolizes a new start. It reminds us that we are liberated from all the mistakes and sorrows that have made our lives so difficult. We are released from the prison that our world and, perhaps more importantly, we have placed us in. We are freed from the regrets and resentments of the past and the fears and expectations of the future. And yes, our timeless spirits are now free from this temporal life and these flawed bodies. Truly, the miracle of Easter is that we get to put all our bad stuff behind us and move forward into a bright new future.

This book has chronicled the unruly System 1 emotions, responses, and dysfunctions that consume our daily lives. We focused on how these seeds over time create bad decisions, unexplainable behaviors, painful relationships, and control issues that ultimately lead to anxiety, guilt, shame, depression, and a deep sense of loneliness. I have also described our extraordinarily complex brains with their numerous parts, complicated wiring, and competing systems of reasoning. It is hard to be human, especially at a time when we are absolutely overwhelmed with situations and information that trigger our most primitive fears, feelings, and behaviors.

I implore you to use the principles in this book to find your journey to freedom so that a year from now you won't wake up on a magnificent Easter morning and catch the rising dawn with another similar set of mistakes, insecurities, regrets, resentments, pains, and sorrows in your heart. The choice to change is yours.

Psychologist Viktor Frankl was a prisoner in four Nazi concentration camps, including Auschwitz, during World War II and lost his wife, mother, and brother in the Holocaust. He wrote, "When we are no longer able to change a situation . . . we are challenged to change ourselves."[12] Every day you remain captive to your System 1 dysfunctions is a day you miss out on freedom.

You opened this book because you understood something in your life had to change. My hope and prayer is that these words were able to push you in a better direction. While you may still be ruminating on the concepts you have learned, I am confident the rewiring process has begun. You stand at the genesis of change. It is up to you to step into the momentum and not look back.

As my son Josh says almost every day, "It's time to quit System 1-ing it!"

Acknowledgments

Thank you:

To God, first and foremost, for his generous love, grace, and guidance. I am humbled that he would use such an imperfect vessel as me to communicate this vital message.

To my coauthors, Margaret Rukstalis and A. J. Gregory. I will always remember and be grateful to my dear friend A. J. for accompanying and guiding me on the most miraculous creative journey I have ever taken.

To Trish, the woman who has captured my heart. You provide great wisdom and help make me a better man. To my inspirational son, Josh, who supported me every day and often every hour during my nine-month journey to write this book. Thank you both from the bottom of my heart.

To my extraordinary other children (Candice, Shane, and Sarah), my beautiful granddaughter (Grace), and Trish's four wonderful children (Adam, Rachel, Donna, and Leah). You have been a constant source of love and inspiration.

To my mom, Ruby, who has always been my biggest fan, my source of strength, and my true north on life's most important issues, as well as to my dad, Floyd (FH), for teaching me life's most significant lessons and most of all how to live free. I miss you every day, Daddy.

To my sisters (Tammy, Tanya, and Debbie) as well as all my incredible nieces and nephews and the entire Chilton family for all your encouragement.

To Dr. Kevin Jung for meeting with me every Friday to shepherd me through complex philosophical issues. To Dr. Ellie Rahbar for helping to edit early versions of the manuscript. To my assistant Denise Griffin Wolfe for keeping it light and me sane through this process.

To my friend and literary agent Esther Fedorkevich and the incredible team, especially Whitney Gossett, at the Fedd Agency.

To Dr. Frank Seekins for your wisdom, support, and care.

To the entire team at Baker, including Chad Allen for believing in the power of this book; Wendy Wetzel and the editorial staff for your artful eye and expertise; and Mark Rice, Hannah Brinks, Eileen Hanson, Brianna DeWitt, and the rest of the marketing and publicity team. We could not have done this without you.

To the literally hundreds of professors I have been blessed to have been trained and mentored by at Western Carolina University, The University of Colorado School of Medicine, Johns Hopkins Medical School, and Wake Forest School of Medicine, and particularly to Drs. Lumb, Wykle, Murphy, Lichtenstein, Undem, and McCall. Thank you for allowing me to stand on your shoulders.

Notes

Introduction

1. *The Wizard of Oz*, directed by Victor Fleming (1939; Culver City, CA: Warner Home Video, 1998), DVD.
2. Paulo Coelho, *Warrior of the Light* (New York: HarperOne, 2003), 15.

Chapter 1 A Tale of Two Minds

1. Charles Dickens, *A Christmas Carol* (New York: Global Classics, 2014), 4.
2. Ibid., 27.
3. B. F. Skinner, *About Behaviorism* (New York: Knopf, 1974); J. Feinberg, *Reason and Responsibility: Readings in Some Basic Problems of Philosophy*, 7th ed. (Belmont, CA: Wadsworth, 1989).
4. See Timothy D. Wilson, *Strangers to Ourselves* (Cambridge, MA: Belknap Press, 2002), 43–44.
5. C. S. Lewis, *The Screwtape Letters* (New York: HarperCollins, 2001), 61.
6. William C. Reeve et al., "Mental Illness Surveillance among Adults in the United States," *Morbidity and Mortality Weekly Report*, September 2, 2011, http://www.cdc.gov/mmwr/preview/mmwrhtml/su6003a1.htm.
7. Ibid.
8. Ibid.

Chapter 2 Stuck in Overdrive

1. Y. Dvir, B. Denietolis, J. A. Frazier, "Childhood Trauma and Psychosis," Child and Adolescent Psychiatric Clinics of North America, October 22, 2014, http://www.ncbi.nlm.nih.gov/pubmed/24012077.

2. Daniel Kahneman, *Thinking, Fast and Slow* (New York: Farrar, Straus and Giroux, 2011).

3. Wilson, *Strangers to Ourselves*, 50.

4. Gary Zukav, *The Seat of the Soul* (New York: Simon & Schuster, 1989), 7.

5. "Embryonic Stem Cells," Science Daily, http://www.sciencedaily.com/terms /embryonic_stem_cell.htm.

6. Tor Nørretranders, *The User Illusion* (New York: Viking, 1998).

7. Kimerer LaMothe, "Emotional Habits: The Key to Addiction," *Psychology Today*, March 16, 2012, https://www.psychologytoday.com/blog/what-body-knows /201203/emotional-habits-the-key-addiction.

Chapter 3 Fear-Obsessed

1. Matthew Weiner, "Smoke Gets in Your Eyes," *Mad Men*, season 1, episode 1, aired July 19, 2007.

2. Martin Lindstrom, *Brandwashed: Tricks Companies Use to Manipulate Our Minds and Persuade Us to Buy* (Great Britain: Kogan Page Limited, 2012), 35.

3. Ibid., 36.

4. Franklin D. Roosevelt, Inaugural Address, March 4, 1933, online at The American Presidency Project by Gerhard Peters and John T. Woolley, http://www .presidency.ucsb.edu/ws/?pid=14473.

5. Lou Dzierzak, "Factoring Fear: What Scares Us and Why," *Scientific American*, October 27, 2008, http://www.scientificamerican.com/article/factor ing-fear-what-scares/.

6. Adapted from http://www.12step.org/docs/Step4_Inventory.pdf.

7. Karl Albrect, "The (Only) 5 Fears We All Share," *Psychology Today*, March 22, 2012, https://www.psychologytoday.com/blog/brainsnacks/201203/the-only -5-fears-we-all-share.

8. Elliot D. Cohen, "The Fear of Losing Control," *Psychology Today*, May 22, 2011, https://www.psychologytoday.com/blog/what-would-aristotle-do/201105 /the-fear-losing-control.

9. Steven Pinker, *The Better Angels of Our Nature: Why Violence Has Declined* (New York: Penguin Books, 2012), 692.

10. Seth Borenstein, "Bombings, Beheadings? Statistics Show a Peaceful World," *Associated Press*, October 23, 2011, http://www.nbcnews.com/id/44999572/ns /world_news/t/bombings-beheadings-statistics-show-peaceful-world/#.VVClWO vVRUS.

11. Steven Pinker, quoted in ibid.

12. John Tierney, "Living in Fear and Paying a High Cost in Heart Risk," *New York Times*, January 15, 2008, http://www.nytimes.com/2008/01/15/science/15tier .html?pagewanted=all.

13. E. Alison Holman, FNP, PhD; Roxane Cohen Silver, PhD; Michael Poulin, PhD; Judith Andersen, PhD; Virginia Gil-Rivas, PhD; Daniel N. McIntosh, PhD, "Terrorism, Acute Stress, and Cardiovascular Health: A 3-Year National Study Following the September 11th Attacks," *Archives of General Psychiatry* 65, no. 1 (2008):73–80, doi:10.1001/archgenpsychiatry.2007.6.

14. William Shakespeare, *Julius Caesar*, act II, scene 2, 32–33.

Chapter 4 Your Brain on Change

1. Aristotle, *Generation of Animals*, trans. A. L. Peck (Cambridge: Harvard University Press, 1979).

2. William James, *The Principles of Psychology*, vol. 1 (New York: Cosimo, 2007), 105.

3. J. S. Griffith and H. R. Mahler, "DNA Ticketing Theory of Memory," *Nature* 223 (1969): 580–82.

4. Norman Doidge, *The Brain That Changes Itself* (New York: Viking, 2007), xv.

5. "I-405 in LA Named Busiest Interstate in Any US City," CBS Los Angeles, August 20, 2013, http://losangeles.cbslocal.com/2013/08/20/i-405-in-la-named -busiest-interstate-in-any-us-city.

6. Doidge, *The Brain That Changes Itself*, 213.

7. "A Logical Proposition (Attributed to Bishop Beckwaith)," *Sunday Critic*, November 22, 1885, http://quoteinvestigator.com/2013/01/10/watch-your-thoughts /#note-5182–4.

8. Elliot Rose, *Experiencing the Soul* (Carlsbad, CA: Hay House, 1998), 15.

9. *Alcoholics Anonymous: The Big Book*, 4th ed. (New York: Alcoholics Anonymous World Services, 2001), 58.

Chapter 5 What It Means to Be Human

1. http://www.oxfordlearnersdictionaries.com/us/definition/english/first-prin ciples.

2. Drake Baer, "Elon Musk Uses This Ancient Critical-Thinking Strategy To Outsmart Everybody Else", Business Insider, January 15, 2015, http://www.busi nessinsider.com/elon-musk-first-principles-2015-1 (accessed January 25, 2016).

3. C. S. Lewis, *The Problem of Pain* (New York: Macmillan, 1962), 127.

4. Erich Fromm, *The Art of Loving* (New York: Harper Perennial Modern Classics, 2006), 9.

5. P. Mellars, "Why Did Modern Human Populations Disperse from Africa ca. 60,000 Years Ago? A New Model," *Proceedings of the National Academy of Sciences* 103 (2006): 9381–9386, doi: 10.1073/pnas.0510792103.

6. R. A. Mathias et al., "Adaptive Evolution of the FADS Gene Cluster within Africa," *PLoS One*, September 19, 2012, 7(9):e44926. doi: 10.1371/journal.pone.0044926.

7. Aaron Smith and Monica Anderson, "5 Facts about Online Dating," *Fact Tank* (blog), Pew Research April 20, 2015, http://www.pewresearch.org/fact-tank /2015/04/20/5-facts-about-online-dating.

8. "New Comscore Social Media User Trends Report," Battenhall, http:// battenhall.net/blog/new-comscore-social-media-user-trends-report.

9. "Mobile Technology Fact Sheet," Pew Research Center, http://www.pew internet.org/fact-sheets/mobile-technology-fact-sheet.

10. "Society's New Addiction: Getting a 'Like' over Having a Life," Vital Smarts, March 12, 2015, https://www.vitalsmarts.com/press/2015/03/societys -new-addiction-getting-a-like-over-having-a-life.

11. Sophie Curtis, "Social Media Users Feel 'Ugly, Inadequate, and Jealous'" *Telegraph*, July 25, 2014, http://www.telegraph.co.uk/technology/social-media /10990297/Social-media-users-feel-ugly-inadequate-and-jealous.html.

12. C. S. Lewis, *The Last Battle* (New York: Collier, 1970), 184.
13. Mother Teresa, *A Simple Path* (New York: Ballantine Books, 1995), 79.

Chapter 6 Right and Wrong Matters

1. Henry Ward Beecher, *Sermons: Henry Ward Beecher, Plymouth Church, Brooklyn*, vol. 2 (New York: Harper & Brothers, 1868), 73.
2. N. T. Wright, *Paul and the Faithfulness of God* (Minneapolis: Fortress Press, 2013), 743.
3. H. G. Frankfurt, "Alternate Possibilities and Moral Responsibility," *Journal of Philosophy* 66, no. 23 (1969): 829–39.
4. E. B. Foa, D. J. Stein, and A. C. McFarlane, "Symptomatology and Psychopathology of Mental Health Problems after Disaster," *Journal of Clinical Psychiatry* 67 (2006): 15–25; O. Agid et al., "Environment and Vulnerability to Major Psychiatric Illness: A Case Control Study of Early Parental Loss in Major Depression, Bipolar Disorder, and Schizophrenia," *Molecular Psychiatry* 4, no. 2 (1999): 163–72.
5. Blaine Harden, foreword to the revised edition of *Escape from Camp 14*, http://www.blaineharden.com.
6. Anderson Cooper, "North Korean Prisoner Escaped after 23 Years," All Things Anderson, December 2, 2012, http://www.allthingsandersoncooper.com/2012/12/anderson-cooper-interviews-shin-dong.html.
7. J. Bryan Lowder, "What Disturbs Us Most about the NY Post Subway Death Cover," *Slate*, December 4, 2012, http://www.slate.com/blogs/behold/2012/12/04/ny_post_subway_death_photo_of_ki_suk_han_why_r_umar_abbasi_s_image_disturbs.html.
8. "The Unethical Rationalization List: 24 and Counting," *Ethics Alarms*, April 14, 2012, http://ethicsalarms.com/2012/04/14/the-unethical-rationalization-list-24-and-counting.

Chapter 7 When Tragedy Strikes

1. Emily Perl Kingsley, "Welcome to Holland," *Our Kids*, 1987, http://www.our-kids.org/archives/Holland.html.
2. Leslie Weatherhead, *The Will of God* (Nashville: Whitmore & Stone, 1944), 12.
3. Ibid.
4. Ibid., 13.
5. Nira Kfir, *Crisis Intervention Verbatim* (New York: Taylor and Francis, 1989), 29.

Chapter 8 Facing the Greatest Challenge—Parenting

1. Erich Fromm, *The Art of Loving* (New York: Harper Perennial Modern Classics, 2006), 36–37.
2. Ibid., 39.
3. Emily Badger, "The Unbelievable Rise of Single Motherhood in America over the Last 50 Years," *Washington Post*, December 18, 2014, http://www

.washingtonpost.com/news/wonkblog/wp/2014/12/18/the-unbelievable-rise-of
-single-motherhood-in-america-over-the-last-50-years.

4. Ron L. Deal, "Marriage, Family, and Stepfamily Statistics," *Smart Step-families*, April 2014, http://www.smartstepfamilies.com/view/statistics.

5. "What Everybody Ought to Know about Narcissism," *Mutual Responsibility*, http://www.mutualresponsibility.org/science/what-everybody-ought-to-know
-about-narcissism.

6. Douglas Belkin, "Today's Anxious Freshmen Declare Majors Far Faster Than Their Elders," *Wall Street Journal*, March 19, 2015, http://www.wsj.com/articles
/todays-anxious-freshmen-declare-majors-far-faster-than-their-elders-1426818334.

Chapter 9 It's Not You, It's Me

1. "Marriage and Divorce in America," Real Relational Solutions, 2007, http://
passionworkshop.com/pdf/marriage_divorce_in_america-FS.pdf.

2. Fromm, *The Art of Loving*, 17.

3. Lisa Firestone, "Differentiation: Living Life on Your Own Terms," *Psychology Today*, November 19, 2009, https://www.psychologytoday.com/blog/com
passion-matters/200911/differentiation-living-life-your-own-terms.

4. Kenneth Levy and J. Wesley Scala, "Transference, Transference Interpreta-tions, and Transference-Focused Psychotherapies," *Psychotherapy* 49, no. 3 (2012): 392, http://www.researchgate.net/profile/J_Scala/publication/230827646_Trans
ference_transference_interpretations_and_transference-focused_psychotherapies
/links/0fcfd506c695cc9c23000000.pdf.

5. Saul McLeod, "Attachment Theory," *Simply Psychology*, 2009, http://www
.simplypsychology.org/attachment.html.

6. George Vaillant, *Triumphs of Experience: The Men of the Harvard Grant Study* (Cambridge, MA: Belknap Press, 2012).

7. Ibid., 113.

8. Ibid., 112–13.

9. Fromm, *The Art of Loving*, 43, 45, 49, 53, 59.

10. Melody Beattie, *Codependent No More: How to Stop Controlling Others and Start Caring for Yourself*, 2nd rev. ed. (Center City: Hazelden, 1992), 36.

11. "Oprah's Life Lesson from Maya Angelou: 'When People Show You Who They Are, Believe Them,'" *Huffington Post*, March 14, 2013, http://www.huffington
post.com/2013/03/14/oprah-life-lesson-maya-angelou_n_2869235.html.

12. Ibid.

Chapter 10 The Gift of Intimacy and Sex

1. Vanessa Taylor, writer, *Hope Springs*, Columbia Pictures, 2012.

2. Helen Fisher, *Why We Love: The Nature and Chemistry of Romantic Love* (New York: Henry Holt, 2004), xv.

3. H. E. Fisher, "Lust, Attraction, and Attachment in Mammalian Reproduc-tion," *Human Nature* (1998): 9, 23–52.

4. David Schnarch, "People Have Sex within the Limits of Their Develop-ment," *Psychology Today*, *Intimacy and Desire* blog, June 4, 2011, https://

www.psychologytoday.com/blog/intimacy-and-desire/201106/people-have-sex
-within-the-limits-their-development.

5. Agustín Fuentes, "Why Is Sex So Complicated?" *Psychology Today*, December 3, 2012, https://www.psychologytoday.com/blog/busting-myths-about
-human-nature/201212/why-is-sex-so-complicated.

6. Helen Fisher, *Anatomy of Love* (New York: Ballantine Books, 1994), 32.

7. David Schnarch, *Intimacy and Desire: Awaken the Passion in Your Relationship* (New York: Beaufort Books, 2009).

8. A. C. Kinsey, W. R. Pomeroy, and C. E. Martin, "Sexual Behavior in the Human Male," *American Journal of Public Health* 93, no. 6 (June 2003): 894–98.

9. "Does Sex Get Better with Age?" MSN Health Hub, August 29, 2014, http://www.msn.com/en-nz/lifestyle/relationships/does-sex-get-better-with-age
/ar-AA5SKMM.

10. "The Allure Aging Survey," *Allure*, http://www.allure.com/beauty-trends
/2013/the-allure-aging-survey?slide=2#slide=1 (accessed January 25, 2016).

11. Stacy Tessler Lindau et al., "A Study of Sexuality and Health among Older Adults in the United States," *New England Journal of Medicine* 357, no. 8 (August 23, 2007): 762–74.

12. Schnarch, *Intimacy and Desire*, 69.

13. William Nicholson, writer, *Shadowlands*, Price Entertainment, 1994.

Chapter 11 Who Am I?

1. Bronnie Ware, *The Top Five Regrets of the Dying: A Life Transformed by the Dearly Departing* (Carlsbad, CA: Hay House, 2012), 37.

2. Christoph Cardinal Schoenborn, *The Joy of Being a Priest: Following the Cure of Ars* (San Francisco: Ignatius Press, 2010), 83.

3. Timothy D. Wilson, *Strangers to Ourselves* (Cambridge, MA: Belknap Press, 2004), 68.

Chapter 12 Surrender

1. Buddy T, "Hitting Bottom," About Health, November 28, 2014, http://
alcoholism.about.com/cs/support/a/aa031997.htm.

2. Ignatius of Loyola, "Suscipe," Loyola Press, http://www.loyolapress.com
/suscipe-prayer-saint-ignatius-of-loyola.htm.

3. "Yoke," Google, https://www.google.com/webhp?sourceid=chrome-instant
&ion=1&espv=2&ie=UTF-8#q=yoke.

4. A. W. Tozer, *I Talk Back to the Devil: The Fighting Fervor of the Victorious Christian* (Camp Hill, PA: First Wingspread Publishers Edition, 2008), Kindle edition.

Chapter 13 Forgiveness and Freedom

1. Nikita Stewart and Richard Perez-Pena, "In Charleston, Raw Emotion at Hearing for Suspect in Church Shooting," *New York Times*, June 19, 2015, http://www.nytimes.com/2015/06/20/us/charleston-shooting-dylann-storm-roof
.html?_r=0.

2. Ibid.

3. "Amish Grandfather: 'We Must Not Think Evil of This Man,'" 2006, http://www.kltv.com/story/5495980/amish-grandfather-we-must-not-think-evil-of-this-man (accessed January 25, 2016).

4. Ibid.

5. Interview with Robert D. Enright about *The Forgiving Life* recorded at the 2011 APA Convention in Washington, DC, American Psychological Association, http://www.apa.org/pubs/books/interviews/4441016-enright.aspx.

6. C. R. Strahan, *The Roan Maverick* (Charleston, SC: Booksurge Publishing, 2006), 162.

7. Martin Luther King Jr. and Coretta Scott King, *A Gift of Love: Sermons from Strength to Love and Other Preachings* (Boston: Beacon Press, 2012), 47.

8. Ibid., 48.

9. See Roy Lloyd and Robert Enright, "The Science of Forgiveness," *Huffington Post*, May 25, 2011, http://www.huffingtonpost.com/roy-lloyd/the-science-of-forgivenes_b_613138.html.

10. Brené Brown, "4 (Totally Surprising) Life Lessons We All Need to Learn," Oprah.com, June 14, 2012, http://www.oprah.com/spirit/Life-Lessons-We-All-Need-to-Learn-Brene-Brown#ixzz3gwXXqr4p.

11. C. S. Lewis, *The Complete C. S. Lewis Signature Classics* (Grand Rapids: Zondervan, 2007), 47–48.

12. Viktor Frankl, *Man's Search for Meaning* (New York: Buccaneer Books, 2006), 116. For more on forgiveness see Roy Lloyd and Robert Enright, "The Science of Forgiveness."

Dr. **Ski Chilton** is a professor in the department of physiology and pharmacology at Wake Forest School of Medicine. He has authored or coauthored more than 130 scientific articles and four books, including *Inflammation Nation*. His work is regularly featured in such venues as WebMD, *Men's Journal*, *Men's Health*, *Prevention*, the *Wall Street Journal*, *ABC News*, and more. He lives in North Carolina.

Dr. **Margaret Rukstalis** is an addiction psychiatrist who has studied the brain and behavior change for over twenty-five years. She received her MD at Dartmouth Medical School, is currently on faculty at Wake Forest School of Medicine, and has coauthored more than fifty scientific articles and book chapters. She lives in North Carolina.

A. J. Gregory is the author of *Messy Faith* and *Silent Savior*. She has also partnered with high-profile figures on over thirty-five memoirs and self-help books, some *New York Times* bestsellers. She lives in New Jersey.

Connect with
DR. SKI

at

DrSkiChilton.com

f Dr. Ski

🐦 @TheDrSki

📷 DrSkiChilton

FREE
Special
Health
Report

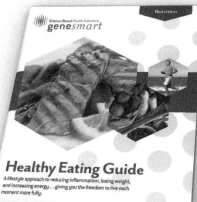
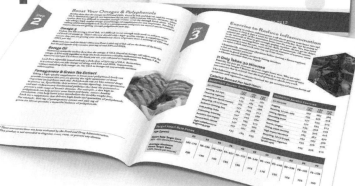
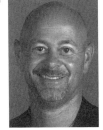

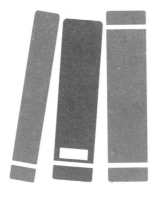

LIKE THIS
BOOK?
Consider sharing
it with others!

- Share or mention the book on your social media platforms. Use the hashtag **#ReWiredBrain**.

- Write a book review on your blog or on a retailer site.

- Pick up a copy for friends, family, or strangers! Anyone who you think would enjoy and be challenged by its message.

- Share this message on Twitter or Facebook. "**I loved #ReWiredBrain by @TheDrSki @ReadBakerBooks**"

- Recommend this book for your church, workplace, book club, or class.

- Follow Baker Books on social media and tell us what you like.

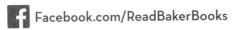 Facebook.com/ReadBakerBooks

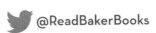 @ReadBakerBooks